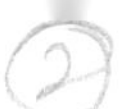

AF333000

HEPATOLOGY RESEARCH AND CLINICAL DEVELOPMENTS

BILE ACIDS

BIOSYNTHESIS, METABOLIC REGULATION AND BIOLOGICAL FUNCTIONS

HEPATOLOGY RESEARCH AND CLINICAL DEVELOPMENTS

Additional books in this series can be found on Nova's website
under the Series tab.

Additional e-books in this series can be found on Nova's website
under the e-book tab.

HEPATOLOGY RESEARCH AND CLINICAL DEVELOPMENTS

BILE ACIDS

BIOSYNTHESIS, METABOLIC REGULATION AND BIOLOGICAL FUNCTIONS

AILEEN MURPHY

EDITOR

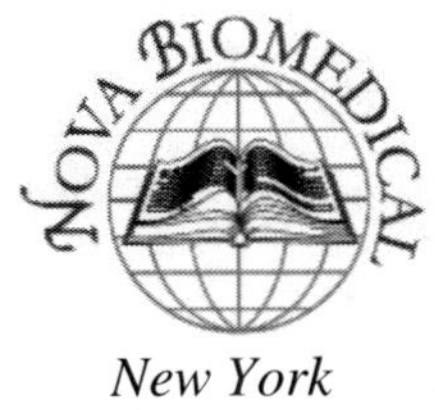

New York

NOTICE TO THE READER

Library of Congress Cataloging-in-Publication Data

ISBN: 978-1-63484-074-3
Library of Congress Control Number: 2015955205

Published by Nova Science Publishers, Inc. † New York

Contents

Preface   **vii**

Chapter 1   The Role of Bile Acids in Different Diseases   **1**
                  Yan-Dong Wang and Wei-Dong Chen

Chapter 2   Bile Acids and Phospholipids Molecular Interaction:
                  From Micells to Mixed Micelles and Biological
                  System   **17**
                  Mihalj Poša and Ana Sebenji

Chapter 3   Bile Aspiration: A Host Factor Modulating Chronic
                  Respiratory Infection   **57**
                  Stephanie Flynn, David F. Woods,
                  Muireann Ní Chróinín, David Mullane,
                  Claire Adams, F. Jerry Reen and Fergal O'Gara

Index   **99**

PREFACE

Bile acids (BAs) have received considerable attention as the key players of systemic metabolism. In the past, bile acids were known to play important roles in absorption of cholesterol, fat-soluble vitamins, and lipids. However, the new roles of bile acids as signaling molecules have been recognized in the last two decades because of discovery of bile acid receptors such as nuclear hormone receptor farnesoid X receptor (FXR) and the membrane receptor G-protein-coupled bile acid receptor 5 (Gpbar1, TGR5). As the metabolic regulators, BAs play pivotal roles in the regulation of bile acid, cholesterol, fatty acid, lipoprotein synthesis, glucose metabolism and energy metabolism. Therefore, BAs, bile acid derivatives, and bile acid sequestrants are potential therapeutic agents for treating a number of metabolic disorders, especially those related to the metabolic syndrome. The first chapter of this book summarizes the basic information of bile acids but focuses on its new functions in different diseases. The next chapter discusses mixed micelles of bile acid salts and phospholipids starting from historical Smalls disc model up to the advanced version as "stacked disk" and "radial shell." The final chapter studies bile aspiration as a host factor for modulating chronic respiratory infection.

Chapter 1 – Bile acids (BAs) have received considerable attention as the key players of systemic metabolism. In the past, bile acids were known to play important roles in absorption of cholesterol, fat-soluble vitamins, and lipids. However, the new roles of bile acids as signaling molecules have been recognized in the last two decades because of discovery of bile acid receptors such as nuclear hormone receptor farnesoid X receptor (FXR) and the membrane receptor G-protein-coupled bile acid receptor 5 (Gpbar1, TGR5). As the metabolic regulators, BAs play pivotal roles in the regulation of bile acid, cholesterol, fatty acid, lipoprotein synthesis, glucose metabolism and energy metabolism. Therefore, BAs, bile acid derivatives, and bile acid sequestrants are potential therapeutic agents for treating a number of metabolic disorders, especially those related to the metabolic syndrome. More recently, the authors' group and others have extended the functions of bile acid receptors FXR and TGR5 to more than metabolic regulation, which include inflammation, liver regeneration, and cancer development. These new findings suggest that bile acids have much broader roles than previously thought, and also highlight bile acids as the therapeutic approach for multiple diseases. This chapter summarizes the basic information of bile acids but focuses on its new functions in different diseases.

Chapter 2 – skeleton. They are mainly synthesized in liver of vertebrates. Bile acid salts form mixed micelles with phospholipids that play important role in transport of cholesterol (i.e., cholesterol is soluble in gallbladder with the help of mixed micelles), as in digestion of lipids in small intestine. Formation of mixed micelles of bile acids and phospholipids is a result of physico- chemical balance between building units in bile canaliculus and kinetic process that involves efflux of bile salts using bile acids protein transporter on basolateral side of hepatocytes. In this chapter, critical discussion is made concerning mixed micelles of bile acid salts and phospholipids starting from historical Smalls disc model up to the advanced version as "stacked disk" and "radial shell". Also, structure of mentioned mixed micelles during incorporation of cholesterol or other different drug molecules is concerned. Binding of bile acids for phospholipids molecules in non micellar environment is discussed as well. This interaction is important in partitioning of bile acid salts in phospholipids bilayer. Molecular and micellar interaction of bile acid salts and phospholipids determines membranotoxicity (membranolytic activity) of bile acids as their promoter role in transport of drugs over membrane lipid barriers, i.e., increasing of membrane permeability (membranolytic activity and permeability of the membrane are directly proportional). Specifically, bile acid oxo derivatives with decreased membranotoxic properties are studied.

Chapter 3 – Bile acid dysmetabolism has long been associated with a broad spectrum of diseases such as diabetes, gastrointestinal disease and obesity (Jones et al. 2014). More recently, however, the aspiration of bile acids into the lungs of respiratory patients has been implicated in the pathophysiology of chronic respiratory disease including cystic fibrosis (CF), chronic obstructive pulmonary disease (COPD) and asthma. Chronic respiratory infections are a leading cause of morbidity and mortality in these patients, particularly in the CF population. Once pathogens have transitioned from an acute to chronic biofilm lifestyle, antibiotic treatments become largely ineffective, severely limiting the clinical management of respiratory diseases. Whilst much is known about the molecular mechanism underpinning this lifestyle switch, little is known about the signals that trigger this detrimental behavioural change. Due to its immense clinical significance it is imperative to identify the signals and pathways responsible for this switch. These subsequently be targeted with novel therapeutic strategies. It has been known for many years that gastro-oesophageal reflux (GOR) is prevalent in the CF. Up to 80% of CF patients exhibit symptoms, with GOR positive patients exhibiting more severe lung disease. Recent evidence suggests that bile, which is refluxed during episodes of GOR, is aspirated into the lungs and is responsible for this observed pathology where it is estimated that aspiration could be as high as 80%. The effectiveness of surgical treatment known as a Nissen fundoplication in controlling progressive lung decline and the limitations of conventional therapies such as proton pump inhibitors supports the role of bile aspiration, not acid reflux underpinning this lung damage. A pervasive microbial signature, strongly dominated by pathogenic proteobacterial species, in the lungs of CF patients has been described with both the biodiversity and community structure correlating with patients disease status and lung function. The lung microbiome in bile aspirating patients was consistent with this pervasive microbial signature, whilst the community profiles of non-aspirating CF patients were consistent with that of healthy non-CF individuals. This is the first evidence implicating aspirated bile in shaping the CF lung microbiome and encouraging disease progression. A possible insight into how this aspirated bile promotes the emergence of pathogenic proteobacteria in the lung comes from recent studies demonstrating the effect of bile on individual respiratory pathogens. The dominant CF pathogen *Pseudomonas aeruginosa*, upregulated phenotypes commonly associated with chronic infection such as biofilm formation and quorum sensing when exposed to bile while phenotypes associated with acute infection were repressed. This further suggests that bile is a major host determinant with a significant role in signaling bacteria to switch to a chronic lifestyle. These new findings, in what is a relatively new and dynamic area of research, hold significant clinical potential for the improvement of both the treatments available and the quality of life of CF patients. It is ultimately hoped that a better understanding of how bile mediates the development of chronic infections can translate into better clinical management of CF.

In: Bile Acids
Editor: Aileen Murphy

ISBN: 978-1-63484-074-3
© 2016 Nova Science Publishers, Inc.

Chapter 1

THE ROLE OF BILE ACIDS IN DIFFERENT DISEASES

Yan-Dong Wang[1], *and Wei-Dong Chen[2],†*

[1]State Key Laboratory of Chemical Resource Engineering,
College of Life Science and Technology, Beijing University
of Chemical Technology, Beijing, P. R. China
[2]Key Laboratory of Receptors-Mediated Gene Regulation
and Drug Discovery, School of Medicine, Henan
University, Kaifeng, Henan, P. R. China

ABSTRACT

Bile acids (BAs) have received considerable attention as the key players of systemic metabolism. In the past, bile acids were known to play important roles in absorption of cholesterol, fat-soluble vitamins, and lipids. However, the new roles of bile acids as signaling molecules have been recognized in the last two decades because of discovery of bile acid receptors such as nuclear hormone receptor farnesoid X receptor (FXR) and the membrane receptor G-protein-coupled bile acid receptor 5 (Gpbar1, TGR5). As the metabolic regulators, BAs play pivotal roles in

* Yan-Dong Wang, PhD: College of Life Science and Technology, Beijing University of Chemical Technology, Beijing, P. R. China. Email: ydwangbuct2009@163.com.
† Wei-Dong Chen, Ph.D. Key Laboratory of Receptors-Mediated Gene Regulation and Drug Discovery, School of Medicine, Henan University, Kaifeng, P. R. China. Email: wdchen666@163.com.

the regulation of bile acid, cholesterol, fatty acid, lipoprotein synthesis, glucose metabolism and energy metabolism. Therefore, BAs, bile acid derivatives, and bile acid sequestrants are potential therapeutic agents for treating a number of metabolic disorders, especially those related to the metabolic syndrome. More recently, our group and others have extended the functions of bile acid receptors FXR and TGR5 to more than metabolic regulation, which include inflammation, liver regeneration, and cancer development. These new findings suggest that bile acids have much broader roles than previously thought, and also highlight bile acids as the therapeutic approach for multiple diseases. This chapter summarizes the basic information of bile acids but focuses on its new functions in different diseases.

INTRODUCTION

Bile acids (BAs) are essential signaling molecules that control various physiological processes such as solubilization of cholesterol in bile, cholesterol elimination, lipid transport, stimulation of bile flow and biliary phospholipid secretion [1, 2]. They also play critical roles in regulation of metabolism in both humans and animal models. In the past, bile acids were known to play important roles in absorption of cholesterol, fat-soluble vitamins, and lipids [3]. However, the new roles of bile acids as signaling molecules have been recognized in the last two decades because of discovery of bile acid receptors such as nuclear hormone receptor farnesoid X receptor (FXR) and the membrane receptor G-protein-coupled bile acid receptor (Gpbar1, TGR5) [4]. As the metabolic regulators, BAs play pivotal roles in the regulation of bile acid, cholesterol, fatty acid, lipoprotein synthesis, glucose metabolism and energy metabolism [5, 6]. Therefore, BAs, bile acid derivatives, and bile acid sequestrants are potential therapeutic agents for treating a number of metabolic disorders, especially those related to the metabolic syndrome [7, 8]. More recently, our group and others have extended the functions of bile acid receptors FXR and TGR5 to more than metabolic regulation, which include inflammation, liver regeneration, and cancer development [1, 4, 9-12]. These new findings suggest that bile acids have much broader roles than previously thought, and also highlight bile acids as the therapeutic approach for multiple diseases.

In this chapter, we will focus on the relation between bile acids and its related cell signaling pathways and the potential for bile acids as a therapeutic approach for obesity, type 2 diabetes (T2D) and cancer.

SYNTHESIS OF BAS

BAs are the end products of cholesterol utilization [13]. It is known that cells utilize several pathways for cholesterol catabolism in mammals. The synthesis of the BAs by enzymes in the liver is the major pathway of cholesterol disposal, which accounts for approximately 90% of cholesterol catabolism [14, 15].

The liver is the only organ where BAs' complete biosynthesis can occur. The synthesis of a full complement of bile acids involves in multiple steps requiring 17 individual enzymes and occurs in multiple intracellular compartments that include endoplasmic reticulum (ER), mitochondria, the cytosol, and peroxisomes [16].

In bile acid synthesis, cytochrome P450s (CYPs) play crucial roles. There are two major pathways for the catabolism of cholesterol to BAs [17]. The pathway via hydroxylation of cholesterol at the 7 position via the action of cholesterol 7α-hydroxylase (CYP7A1) is the classic ('neutral') pathway of bile acid synthesis. The classic pathway in humans leads to the biosynthesis of two primary BAs, cholic acid (CA) and chenodeoxycholic acid (CDCA), which are the most abundant in human bile (CDCA (45%)) and (CA (31%)) [18]. CYP7A1 is the rate-limiting enzyme of the classic pathway.

There is an alternative pathway that involves oxidation of cholesterol at the 27 position by the mitochondrial enzyme sterol 27-hydroxylase (CYP27A1), which is subsequently hydroxylated by oxysterol 7α-hydroxylase (CYP7B1). This alternative pathway is regarded as the "acidic" pathway of bile acid synthesis.

Primary bile acids such as CA and CDCA are synthesized in the liver. After synthesis, these BAs are conjugated via an amide bond at the terminal carboxyl group with glycine or taurine. These conjugation reactions yield glycoconjugates and tauroconjugates, respectively. Conjugated primary bile acids include glycocholic acid and taurocholic acid (derivatives of cholic acid), glycohenodeoxycholic acid and taurochenodeoxycholic acid (derivatives of chenodeoxycholic acid) [19]. They are the major bile salts in bile and are roughly equal in concentration. The conjugated BAs are excreted and stored in the gall bladder.

In humans, 95% of BAs are reabsorbed in the terminal ileum and less than 5% of the BA pool enters the colon per day. Secondary bile acids result from bacterial actions in the colon. The primary BAs (CA and CDCA) that enter the colon are metabolized by bacterial flora and converted into the secondary BAs, DCA and LCA, respectively [20].

SIGNALING PATHWAYS RELATED TO BAS

BAs, serving as signaling molecules, have various direct metabolic actions in the body through the nuclear receptor Farnesoid X receptor (FXR) and the G protein-coupled bile acid receptor 1 (Gpbar1 or TGR5). Many of their functions as signaling molecules in the liver and the intestines are by activating FXR, whereas TGR5 may be involved in metabolic, endocrine and neurological functions [3]. Moreover, BAs can activate cell signaling pathways (c-jun N-terminal kinase 1/2, AKT, and ERK1/2) involved in the regulation of the pathogenesis of BA-associated lung injury and apoptosis [15, 21, 22].

The Nuclear Bile Acid Receptor FXR

BAs, in particular CDCA and CA, can regulate the expression of genes involved in their synthesis through activating FXR. FXR is the primary sensor of BAs. The FXRs belong to the superfamily of nuclear receptors that includes the steroid/thyroid hormone receptor family as well as the liver X receptors (LXRs), retinoid X receptors (RXRs), and the peroxisome proliferator-activated receptors (PPARs) [1, 2]. As a metabolic regulator, FXR plays key roles in bile acid, cholesterol, lipid, and glucose metabolism. Therefore, FXR is a potential drug target for a number of metabolic disorders, especially those related to the metabolic syndrome. More recently, our group and others have extended the functions of FXR to more than metabolic regulation, which include anti-bacterial growth in intestine, liver regeneration, and hepatocarcinogenesis [9-11]. These new findings suggest that FXR has much broader roles than previously thought, and also highlight FXR as a drug target for multiple diseases.

The function of FXR has been shown to be related to different diseases including cholestasis, diabetes, atherosclerosis, and cholesterol gallstone disease. FXR fulfills its regulatory role by controlling the expression of a variety of genes in cognate metabolic pathways. By binding to FXREs, FXR regulates many genes belonging to different metabolic pathways (Figure 1). Activation of FXR alters the expression of different groups of genes involved in BA homoeostasis, lipid metabolism, glucose balance and liver regeneration. FXR activates the expression of short heterodimer partner (SHP), which in turn binds to and inactivates liver receptor homolog 1 (LRH-1, NR5A2), thus potently inhibiting the expression of cholesterol 7α-hydroxylase (CYP7A1), the rate-limiting enzyme in BA biosynthesis [23]. In addition, it is clear that BA activation of FXR in the intestine leads to the induction of mouse Fgf15 [24] or its human ortholog FGF19 [25], thereby suppressing CYP7A1 expression through a JNK-dependent signaling cascade. The recent report shows that FXR activates MAFG to suppress bile acid synthesis and metabolism [26]. FXR also activates the expression of hepatic Insig-2, which represses cholesterol synthesis [27]. These findings indicate that FXR not only directly suppresses the synthesis of BAs, but also inhibits the synthesis of cholesterol, the precursor for BAs. A constant pool of BAs was maintained by enterohepatic circulation. In addition to regulating BA synthesis, FXR controls the recycling of BAs by regulating genes involved in BA secretion, transportation, absorption, conjugation, and detoxification [28, 29]. The remarkable ability of FXR to regulate BA metabolism is confirmed by loss-of-function studies on FXR in animal model [30, 31].

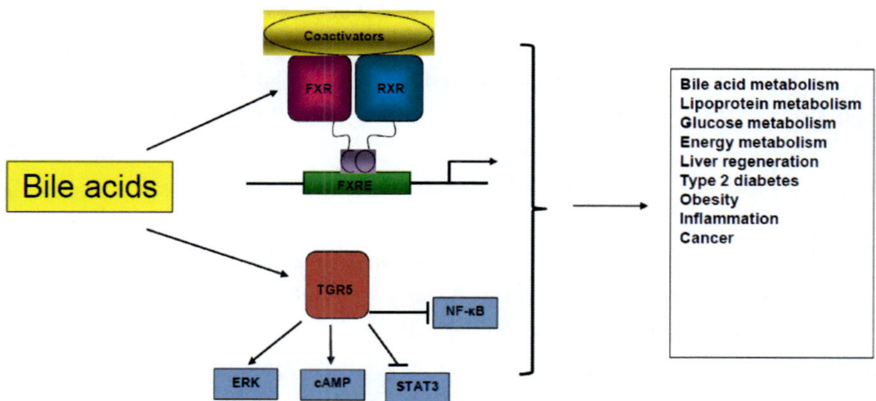

Figure 1. BAs are related to different diseases through FXR and TGR5. FXR activation by BAs regulates bile acid metabolism, lipoprotein metabolism and glucose metabolism through regulating various target genes. FXR is a regulator in different diseases such as liver regeneration, type 2 diabetes, inflammation and cancer. TGR5 activation by BAs regulates lipoprotein metabolism, glucose metabolism and energy metabolism. TGR5 may be a potential suppressor in type 2 diabetes, obesity, inflammation, and cancer through regulation of cAMP, NF-κB, STAT3 and other cell signaling.

Therefore, FXR is also called the BA receptor due to its master effect on BA homeostasis. Analyses of FXR knockout animals also reveal an unexpected role of FXR in lipid metabolism. It was shown that FXR also regulates a set of genes that participate in lipoprotein metabolism. These include genes for PLTP, SDC-1, the very low density lipoprotein receptor

(VLDLR), apolipoprotein C-II, and apolipoprotein E [32-34]. These genes are involved in the metabolism of plasma lipoproteins. In addition, activation of FXR leads to repression of SREBP-1c, a transcription factor that controls genes involved in fatty acid and triglyceride synthesis [35-37]. Therefore, FXR plays an important role in regulating lipid metabolism. Because of the intrinsic interaction between lipid and glucose metabolism, it was not surprising to find that FXR was also involved in the regulation of glucose levels. FXR regulates gene expression of phosphoenolpyruvate carboxykinase (PEPCK) [38], which is a key enzyme of the hepatic gluconeogenesis pathway, by catalyzing a critical step in gluconeogenesis.

The Membrane Bile Acid Receptor TGR5

TGR5 as a bile acid receptor was found in 2002 [39]. High levels of TGR5 mRNA were detected in several tissues such as small intestine, stomach, liver, lung, especially in placenta and spleen [40]. As a GPCR, TGR5 can be activated by bile acids, inducing the production of cAMP [39]. Typically, TGR5 is located at the plasma membrane. But it is internalized into the cytoplasm in response to its agonists [41]. TGR5 is connected with several cell signaling and diseases. TGR5 plays important roles in cell signaling such as NF-κB [42], AKT [43] and ERK [44]. TGR5 agonists have been studied to be used in treatments of metabolic, inflammatory and digestive disorders [45].

Our group identified TGR5 negatively regulates hepatic inflammatory response through antagonizing NF-κB [12]. We found TGR5 activation suppressed the phosphorylation of IκBα, the translocation of p65, NF-κB DNA binding activity and its transcription activity in HepG2 cells. Furthermore, the activation of TGR5 enhanced the interaction of IκBα and β-arrestin2. This interaction suppressed NF-κB transcription activity [42]. In the same year, Pols et al. found TGR5 activation with INT-777 decreased nuclear translocation of p65 and phosphorylation of IκBα in macrophages [46]. Our group found that TGR5 was a suppressor of gastric cancer cell proliferation and migration through antagonizing STAT3 signaling pathway [47]. TGR5 activation antagonized STAT3 signaling pathway through suppressing the phosphorylation of STAT3 and its transcription activity induced by lipoplysaccharide (LPS) or IL-6. TGR5 overexpression with ligand treatment inhibited gene expression mediated by STAT3.

It suggests that TGR5 antagonizes gastric cancer proliferation and migration at least in part by inhibiting STAT3 signaling. These findings identify TGR5 as an attractive therapeutic tool for human gastric cancer [47].

Other Signaling Pathways

BAs are also related to other signaling pathways such as JNK1/2, ERK1/2, and PERK-eIF2α-ATF4 signaling. For example, Su et al. reported that CDCA induced significant p38 and c-Jun N-terminal kinase (JNK) phosphorylation, cytosolic phospholipase A2 (cPLA2) and cyclooxygenase-2 (COX-2) messenger RNA expression, PGE2 production, which may contribute to the pathogenesis of BA-associated lung injury [14]. Taurolithocholic acid promotes intrahepatic cholangiocarcinoma cell growth via muscarinic acetylcholine receptor and EGFR/ERK1/2 signaling pathway [48].

Tauroursodeoxycholic acid attenuates inorganic phosphate-induced osteoblastic differentiation and mineralization in NIH3T3 fibroblasts by inhibiting the ER stress response PERK-eIF2α-ATF4 pathway [49]. Broeders et al. reported that CDCA increases human brown adipose tissue activity through increasing mitochondrial uncoupling and D2 expression [50].

THE FUNCTIONS OF BAS IN DIFFERENT DISEASES

BAs and Type 2 Diabetes

Diabetes is a kind of endocrine diseases, characterized by hyperglycemia. It is a growing health problem in the world, and may lead cause of death, but the currently available strategies for therapy and prevention are insufficient. Recent observations indicate that bile acid homeostasis is altered in type 2 diabetes (T2D). In the early 1990s, it was observed that bile acid sequestrants improved glycaemic control in patients with T2D. BA sequestrants have been approved in the US for the treatment of T2D. Now it is known that BAs are the natural ligands of both FXR and TGR5, contributing to regulation of glucose metabolism. FXR regulates gene expression of phosphoenolpyruvate carboxykinase (PEPCK) [38], which is a key enzyme of the hepatic gluconeogenesis pathway, by catalyzing a critical step in gluconeogenesis. Activation of FXR in wild-type or diabetic [db/db or KKA-(y)] mice promotes hypoglycemia and increases insulin sensitivity.

TGR5, as a bile acid membrane receptor, is reported that its activation could promote glucagon-like peptide-1 (GLP-1) secretion in a murine enteroendocrine cell line STC-1 [51]. GLP-1 can increase insulin secretion from the pancreas in a glucose-dependent manner, increase insulin-sensitivity in both alpha cells and beta cells, and increase beta cells mass and insulin expression to regulate glucose metabolism. So BAs have regulation actions in T2D, acting through FXR and TGR5.

BAs and Obesity

Obesity becomes great threat to public health in the whole world. The energy intake exceeds expenditure, resulting in obesity. It is known that brown adipose tissue (BAT) plays key roles for prevention and treatment of obesity through dissipating energy as heat by thermogenesis [52]. BAT is compared of thermogenic adipocytes, converting chemical energy to heat. Because of the key role of BAT in energy burning, BAT is considered to combat obesity. Increase of activity of BAT is an easy way to increase energy burning. It is found that the administration of BAs to mice can increase the energy expenditure in BAT. This effect results in activation of TGR5. And it is not connected with FXR [52]. The activation of TGR5 increases the level of cAMP-dependent thyroid hormone-activating enzyme, type 2 iodothyronine deiodinase (D2). D2 is one of major thermogenic protein. It can convert thyroxine (T4) to active tri-iodothyronine (T3) in BAT. Bile acids treatment in BAT and human skeletal muscle cells increases D2 activity, oxygen consumption and extracellular acidification rate [36]. Recent study also found bile acid CDCA had effect on human BAT activity. Treatment of 12 healthy female subjects with CDCA for 2 days results in increasing BAT activity [53]. It suggests that BAs are important regulators in obesity.

BAs and Cancer

BAs are endogenous agents capable of causing cancer throughout the gastrointestinal (GI) tract. BA induces an increase in the gene expression of COX-2 via the sequential transcriptional induction of SHP and CDX1 in precancerous lesions of human gastric cancer [54]. Mariette et al. reported that BAs, as tumour promoters, up-regulate MUC4 expression to promote tumor progression [55]. BAs may also have some importance in the development of colorectal cancer [56, 57].

Deoxycholic acid (DCA) is increased in the colonic contents of humans in response to a high fat diet. In populations with a high incidence of colorectal cancer, fecal concentrations of BAs are higher, and this association suggests that increased colonic exposure to BAs could play a role in the development of cancer. Elevated BA levels also increase hepatocellular carcinoma. Anakk et al. reported that mice with a severe defect in BA homeostasis due to the loss of the nuclear receptors FXR and SHP have enlarged livers, progenitor cell proliferation, and Yes-associated protein (YAP) activation and develop spontaneous liver tumorigenesis. BAs act as upstream regulators of YAP via a pathway dependent on the induction of the scaffold protein IQGAP1. Patients with diverse biliary dysfunctions exhibit enhanced IQGAP1 and nuclear YAP expression. The findings reveal the mechanism for BA regulation of liver growth and tumorigenesis via the Hippo pathway [58].

PROSPECTS

The function of BAs is expanded rapidly from initial roles in helping lipid digestion and absorption due to the discovery of FXR and TGR5. As the natural ligands of FXR and TGR5, BAs suppress inflammation, regulate glucose, energy and lipid metabolism. At the same time, BAs are inherently toxic compounds due to the induction of liver and lung injury. Therefore, BAs are important cell regulators. Currently, new BA agonists and antagonists are being developed for therapeutic purposes. We expect that further investigation of BA function in these new areas will provide novel insights into the complex mechanism of BAs in metabolism and different diseases.

ACKNOWLEDGMENTS

We apologize to colleagues whose work could not be cited due to space limitations. Yan-Dong Wang is supported by the National Natural Science Foundation of China (Grant No. 81370537) and the Fundamental Research Funds for the Central Universities (Grant No. YS1407 and 2050205).

Wei-Dong Chen is supported by the National Natural Science Foundation of China (Grant No. 81270522 and Grant No. 81472232), Program for Science and Technology Innovation Talents in Universities of Henan Province (HASTIT, Grant No. 13HASTIT024) and Plan for Scientific Innovation Talent of Henan Province.

REFERENCES

[1]   Wang, Y. D., Chen, W. D. and Huang, W. 2008. FXR, a target for different diseases. *Histol. Histopathol.* 23:621-627.

[2]   Wang, Y. D., Chen, W. D., Moore, D. D. and Huang, W. 2008. FXR: a metabolic regulator and cell protector. *Cell Res.* 18:1087-1095.

[3]   Ma, H. and Patti, M. E. 2014. Bile acids, obesity, and the metabolic syndrome. *Best Pract. Res. Clin. Gastroenterol.* 28:573-583.

[4]   Wang, Y. D., Chen, W. D., Wang, M., Yu, D., Forman, B. M. and Huang, W. 2008. Farnesoid X receptor antagonizes nuclear factor kappaB in hepatic inflammatory response. *Hepatology* 48:1632-1643.

[5]   Sonne, D. P., Hansen, M. and Knop, F. K. 2014. Bile acid sequestrants in type 2 diabetes: potential effects on GLP1 secretion. *Eur. J. Endocrinol.* 171:R47-65.

[6]   Boesjes, M. and Brufau, G. 2014. Metabolic effects of bile acids in the gut in health and disease. *Curr. Med. Chem.* 21:2822-2829.

[7]   Pols, T. W., Noriega, L. G., Nomura, M., Auwerx, J. and Schoonjans, K. 2011. The bile acid membrane receptor TGR5 as an emerging target in metabolism and inflammation. *J. Hepatol.* 54:1263-1272.

[8]   Miyazaki-Anzai, S., Masuda, M., Levi, M., Keenan, A. L. and Miyazaki, M. 2014. Dual activation of the bile acid nuclear receptor FXR and G-protein-coupled receptor TGR5 protects mice against atherosclerosis. *PLoS One* 9:e108270.

[9]   Chen, W. D., Wang, Y. D., Zhang, L., Shiah, S., Wang, M., Yang, F., Yu, D., Forman, B. M. and Huang, W. 2010. Farnesoid X receptor alleviates age-related proliferation defects in regenerating mouse livers by activating forkhead box m1b transcription. *Hepatology* 51:953-962.

[10]   Wang, Y. D., Chen, W. D., Li, C., Guo, C., Li, Y., Qi, H., Shen, H., Kong, J., Long, X., Yuan, F. et al. 2015. Farnesoid X Receptor Antagonizes JNK Signaling Pathway in Liver Carcinogenesis by Activating SOD3. *Mol. Endocrinol.* 29:322-331.

[11]   Wang, Y. D., Yang, F., Chen, W. D., Huang, X., Lai, L., Forman, B. M. and Huang, W. 2008. Farnesoid X receptor protects liver cells from

apoptosis induced by serum deprivation in vitro and fasting in vivo. *Mol. Endocrinol.* 22:1622-1632.

[12] Wang, Y. D., Chen, W. D., Yu, D., Forman, B. M. and Huang, W. 2011. The G-protein-coupled bile acid receptor, Gpbar1 (TGR5), negatively regulates hepatic inflammatory response through antagonizing nuclear factor kappa light-chain enhancer of activated B cells (NF-kappaB) in mice. *Hepatology* 54:1421-1432.

[13] Kuipers, F., Bloks, V. W. and Groen, A. K. 2014. Beyond intestinal soap--bile acids in metabolic control. *Nat. Rev. Endocrinol.* 10:488-498.

[14] Su, K. C., Wu, Y. C., Chen, C. S., Hung, M. H., Hsiao, Y. H., Tseng, C. M., Chang, S. C., Lee, Y. C. and Perng, D. W. 2013. Bile acids increase alveolar epithelial permeability via mitogen-activated protein kinase, cytosolic phospholipase A2, cyclooxygenase-2, prostaglandin E2 and junctional proteins. *Respirology* 18:848-856.

[15] Klaassen, C. D. and Cui, J. Y. 2015. Review: Mechanisms of How the Intestinal Microbiota Alters the Effects of Drugs and Bile Acids. *Drug Metab. Dispos.* 43:1505-1521.

[16] Barrera, F., Azocar, L., Molina, H., Schalper, K. A., Ocares, M., Liberona, J., Villarroel, L., Pimentel, F., Perez-Ayuso, R. M., Nervi, F. et al. 2015. Effect of cholecystectomy on bile acid synthesis and circulating levels of fibroblast growth factor 19. *Ann. Hepatol.* 14:710-721.

[17] Li, T. and Apte, U. 2015. Bile Acid Metabolism and Signaling in Cholestasis, Inflammation, and Cancer. *Adv. Pharmacol.* 74:263-302.

[18] Mazuy, C., Helleboid, A., Staels, B. and Lefebvre, P. 2015. Nuclear bile acid signaling through the farnesoid X receptor. *Cell. Mol. Life Sci.* 72: 1631-1650.

[19] Tian, J., Keller, M. P., Oler, A. T., Rabaglia, M. E., Schueler, K. L., Stapleton, D. S., Broman, A. T., Zhao, W., Kendziorski, C., Yandell, B. S. et al. 2015. Identification of the Bile Transporter Slco1a6 as a Candidate Gene that Broadly Affects Gene Expression in Mouse Pancreatic Islets. *Genetics.*

[20] Changbumrung, S., Tungtrongchitr, R., Migasena, P. and Chamroenngan, S. 1990. Serum unconjugated primary and secondary bile acids in patients with cholangiocarcinoma and hepatocellular carcinoma. *J. Med. Assoc. Thai.* 73:81-90.

[21] Abdel-Latif, M. M., Inoue, H. and Reynolds, J. V. 2015. Opposing effects of bile acids deoxycholic acid and ursodeoxycholic acid on signal transduction pathways in oesophageal cancer cells. *Eur. J. Cancer Prev.*

[22] Amaral, J. D., Viana, R. J., Ramalho, R. M., Steer, C. J. and Rodrigues, C.M. 2009. Bile acids: regulation of apoptosis by ursodeoxycholic acid. *J. Lipid Res.* 50:1721-1734.

[23] Li, T. and Chiang, J. Y. 2015. Bile acids as metabolic regulators. *Curr. Opin. Gastroenterol.* 31:159-165.

[24] Modica, S., Petruzzelli, M., Bellafante, E., Murzilli, S., Salvatore, L., Celli, N., Di Tullio, G., Palasciano, G., Moustafa, T., Halilbasic, E. et al. 2012. Selective activation of nuclear bile acid receptor FXR in the intestine protects mice against cholestasis. *Gastroenterology* 142:355-365 e351-354.

[25] Miyata, M., Hata, T., Yamazoe, Y. and Yoshinari, K. 2014. SREBP-2 negatively regulates FXR-dependent transcription of FGF19 in human intestinal cells. *Biochem. Biophys. Res. Commun.* 443:477-482.

[26] de Aguiar Vallim, T. Q., Tarling, E. J., Ahn, H., Hagey, L. R., Romanoski, C. E., Lee, R. G., Graham, M. J., Motohashi, H., Yamamoto, M. and Edwards, P. A. 2015. MAFG is a transcriptional repressor of bile acid synthesis and metabolism. *Cell Metab.* 21:298-310.

[27] Hubbert, M. L., Zhang, Y., Lee, F. Y. and Edwards, P.A. 2007. Regulation of hepatic Insig-2 by the farnesoid X receptor. *Mol. Endocrinol.* 21:1359-1369.

[28] Ananthanarayanan, M., Balasubramanian, N., Makishima, M., Mangelsdorf, D. J. and Suchy, F.J. 2001. Human bile salt export pump promoter is transactivated by the farnesoid X receptor/bile acid receptor. *J. Biol. Chem.* 276:28857-28865.

[29] Kast, H. R., Goodwin, B., Tarr, P. T., Jones, S. A., Anisfeld, A. M., Stoltz, C. M., Tontonoz, P., Kliewer, S., Willson, T. M. and Edwards, P. A. 2002. Regulation of multidrug resistance-associated protein 2 (ABCC2) by the nuclear receptors pregnane X receptor, farnesoid X-activated receptor, and constitutive androstane receptor. *J. Biol. Chem.* 277:2908-2915.

[30] Sinal, C. J., Tohkin, M., Miyata, M., Ward, J. M., Lambert, G. and Gonzalez, F. J. 2000. Targeted disruption of the nuclear receptor FXR/BAR impairs bile acid and lipid homeostasis. *Cell* 102:731-744.

[31] Kok, T., Hulzebos, C. V., Wolters, H., Havinga, R., Agellon, L. B., Stellaard, F., Shan, B., Schwarz, M. and Kuipers, F. 2003. Enterohepatic circulation of bile salts in farnesoid X receptor-deficient mice: efficient intestinal bile salt absorption in the absence of ileal bile acid-binding protein. *J. Biol. Chem.* 278:41930-41937.

[32] Edwards, P. A., Kast, H. R. and Anisfeld, A. M. 2002. BAREing it all: the adoption of LXR and FXR and their roles in lipid homeostasis. *J. Lipid Res.* 43:2-12.

[33] Anisfeld, A. M., Kast-Woelbern, H. R., Lee, H., Zhang, Y., Lee, F. Y. and Edwards, P. A. 2005. Activation of the nuclear receptor FXR induces fibrinogen expression: a new role for bile acid signaling. *J. Lipid Res.* 46:458-468.

[34] Sirvent, A., Claudel, T., Martin, G., Brozek, J., Kosykh, V., Darteil, R., Hum, D. W., Fruchart, J. C. and Staels, B. 2004. The farnesoid X receptor induces very low density lipoprotein receptor gene expression. *FEBS Lett.* 566:173-177.

[35] Zhang, Y., Castellani, L. W., Sinal, C. J., Gonzalez, F. J. and Edwards, P. A. 2004. Peroxisome proliferator-activated receptor-gamma coactivator 1alpha (PGC-1alpha) regulates triglyceride metabolism by activation of the nuclear receptor FXR. *Genes Dev.* 18:157-169.

[36] Watanabe, M., Houten, S. M., Mataki, C., Christoffolete, M. A., Kim, B. W., Sato, H., Messaddeq, N., Harney, J. W., Ezaki, O., Kodama, T. et al. 2006. Bile acids induce energy expenditure by promoting intracellular thyroid hormone activation. *Nature* 439:484-489.

[37] Watanabe, M., Houten, S. M., Wang, L., Moschetta, A., Mangelsdorf, D. J., Heyman, R. A., Moore, D. D. and Auwerx, J. 2004. Bile acids lower triglyceride levels via a pathway involving FXR, SHP, and SREBP-1c. *J. Clin. Invest.* 113:1408-1418.

[38] Stayrook, K. R., Bramlett, K. S., Savkur, R. S., Ficorilli, J., Cook, T., Christe, M. E., Michael, L. F. and Burris, T. P. 2005. Regulation of carbohydrate metabolism by the farnesoid X receptor. *Endocrinology* 146:984-991.

[39] Maruyama, T., Miyamoto, Y., Nakamura, T., Tamai, Y., Okada, H., Sugiyama, E., Nakamura, T., Itadani, H. and Tanaka, K. 2002. Identification of membrane-type receptor for bile acids (M-BAR). *Biochem. Biophys. Res. Commun.* 298:714-719.

[40] Tiwari, A. and Maiti, P. 2009. TGR5: an emerging bile acid G-protein-coupled receptor target for the potential treatment of metabolic disorders. *Drug Discov. Today* 14:523-530.

[41] Kawamata, Y., Fujii, R., Hosoya, M., Harada, M., Yoshida, H., Miwa, M., Fukusumi, S., Habata, Y., Itoh, T., Shintani, Y. et al. 2003. A G protein-coupled receptor responsive to bile acids. *J. Biol. Chem.* 278: 9435-9440.

[42] Meng, Z., Liu, N., Fu, X., Wang, X., Wang, Y. D., Chen, W. D., Zhang, L., Forman, B. M. and Huang, W. 2011. Insufficient bile acid signaling impairs liver repair in CYP27(-/-) mice. *J. Hepatol.* 55:885-895.

[43] Kida, T., Tsubosaka, Y., Hori, M., Ozaki, H. and Murata, T. 2013. Bile acid receptor TGR5 agonism induces NO production and reduces monocyte adhesion in vascular endothelial cells. *Arterioscler. Thromb. Vasc. Biol.* 33:1663-1669.

[44] Masyuk, A. I., Huang, B. Q., Radtke, B. N., Gajdos, G. B., Splinter, P. L., Masyuk, T. V., Gradilone, S. A. and LaRusso, N. F. 2013. Ciliary subcellular localization of TGR5 determines the cholangiocyte functional response to bile acid signaling. *Am. J. Physiol. Gastrointest. Liver Physiol.* 304:G1013-1024.

[45] Fan, M., Wang, X., Xu, G., Yan, Q. and Huang, W. 2015. Bile acid signaling and liver regeneration. *Biochim. Biophys. Acta* 1849:196-200.

[46] Pols, T. W., Nomura, M., Harach, T., Lo Sasso, G., Oosterveer, M. H., Thomas, C., Rizzo, G., Gioiello, A., Adorini, L., Pellicciari, R. et al. 2011. TGR5 activation inhibits atherosclerosis by reducing macrophage inflammation and lipid loading. *Cell Metab.* 14:747-757.

[47] Guo, C. S. J. L., Z.; Xiao, R., Wen, J., Li, Y., Zhang, M., Zhang, X., Yu, D., Huang,W., Chen,W.-D., Wang, Y.-D. 2015. The G-protein-coupled bile acid receptor Gpbar1 (TGR5) suppresses gastric cancer cell proliferation and migration through antagonizing STAT3 signaling pathway. *Oncotarget.*

[48] Amonyingcharoen, S., Suriyo, T., Thiantanawat, A., Watcharasit, P. and Satayavivad, J. 2015. Taurolithocholic acid promotes intrahepatic cholangiocarcinoma cell growth via muscarinic acetylcholine receptor and EGFR/ERK1/2 signaling pathway. *Int. J. Oncol.* 46:2317-2326.

[49] Liu, F., Cui, Y., Ge, P., Luan, J., Zhou, X. and Han, J. 2015. Tauroursodeoxycholic acid attenuates inorganic phosphate-induced osteoblastic differentiation and mineralization in NIH3T3 fibroblasts by inhibiting the ER stress response PERK-eIF2alpha-ATF4 pathway. *Drug Discov. Ther.* 9:38-44.

[50] Broeders, E. P., Nascimento, E. B., Havekes, B., Brans, B., Roumans, K. H., Tailleux, A., Schaart, G., Kouach, M., Charton, J., Deprez, B. et al. 2015. The Bile Acid Chenodeoxycholic Acid Increases Human Brown Adipose Tissue Activity. *Cell Metab.* 22:418-426.

[51] Katsuma, S., Hirasawa, A. and Tsujimoto, G. 2005. Bile acids promote glucagon-like peptide-1 secretion through TGR5 in a murine

enteroendocrine cell line STC-1. *Biochem. Biophys. Res. Commun.* 329: 386-390.

[52] Chen, X., Lou, G., Meng, Z. and Huang, W. 2011. TGR5: a novel target for weight maintenance and glucose metabolism. *Exp. Diabetes Res.* 2011:853501.

[53] Broeders, E. P., Nascimento, E. B., Havekes, B., Brans, B., Roumans, K. H., Tailleux, A., Schaart, G., Kouach, M., Charton, J., Deprez, B. et al. 2015. The Bile Acid Chenodeoxycholic Acid Increases Human Brown Adipose Tissue Activity. *Cell Metab.*

[54] Park, M. J., Kim, K. H., Kim, H. Y., Kim, K. and Cheong, J. 2008. Bile acid induces expression of COX-2 through the homeodomain transcription factor CDX1 and orphan nuclear receptor SHP in human gastric cancer cells. *Carcinogenesis* 29:2385-2393.

[55] Mariette, C., Perrais, M., Leteurtre, E., Jonckheere, N., Hemon, B., Pigny, P., Batra, S., Aubert, J. P., Triboulet, J. P. and Van Seuningen, I. 2004. Transcriptional regulation of human mucin MUC4 by bile acids in oesophageal cancer cells is promoter-dependent and involves activation of the phosphatidylinositol 3-kinase signalling pathway. *Biochem. J.* 377:701-708.

[56] Zeng, H., Claycombe, K. J. and Reindl, K. M. 2015. Butyrate and deoxycholic acid play common and distinct roles in HCT116 human colon cell proliferation. *J. Nutr. Biochem.*

[57] Zhu, Y., Zhu, M. and Lance, P. 2012. Stromal COX-2 signaling activated by deoxycholic acid mediates proliferation and invasiveness of colorectal epithelial cancer cells. *Biochem. Biophys. Res. Commun.* 425: 607-612.

[58] Anakk, S., Bhosale, M., Schmidt, V. A., Johnson, R. L., Finegold, M. J. and Moore, D. D. 2013. Bile acids activate YAP to promote liver carcinogenesis. *Cell Rep.* 5:1060-1069.

In: Bile Acids
Editor: Aileen Murphy

ISBN: 978-1-63484-074-3
© 2016 Nova Science Publishers, Inc.

Chapter 2

BILE ACIDS AND PHOSPHOLIPIDS MOLECULAR INTERACTION: FROM MICELLS TO MIXED MICELLES AND BIOLOGICAL SYSTEM

Mihalj Poša and Ana Sebenji*

Department of Pharmacy, Faculty of Medicine,
University of Novi Sad, Autonomous Province of Vojvodina, Serbia

ABSTRACT

Bile acids are amphiphiles, surface active compounds with steroid skeleton. They are mainly synthesized in liver of vertebrates. Bile acid salts form mixed micelles with phospholipids that play important role in transport of cholesterol (i.e., cholesterol is soluble in gallbladder with the help of mixed micelles), as in digestion of lipids in small intestine. Formation of mixed micelles of bile acids and phospholipids is a result of physico- chemical balance between building units in bile canaliculus and kinetic process that involves efflux of bile salts using bile acids protein transporter on basolateral side of hepatocytes. In this chapter, critical discussion is made concerning mixed micelles of bile acid salts and phospholipids starting from historical Smalls disc model up to the advanced version as "stacked disk" and "radial shell". Also, structure of

---

* Author to whom correspondence should be addressed; E-Mail: mihaljp@uns.ac.rs Tel.: +381-63-11-400-15.

mentioned mixed micelles during incorporation of cholesterol or other different drug molecules is concerned. Binding of bile acids for phospholipids molecules in non micellar environment is discussed as well. This interaction is important in partitioning of bile acid salts in phospholipids bilayer. Molecular and micellar interaction of bile acid salts and phospholipids determines membranotoxicity (membranolytic activity) of bile acids as their promoter role in transport of drugs over membrane lipid barriers, i.e., increasing of membrane permeability (membranolytic activity and permeability of the membrane are directly proportional). Specifically, bile acid oxo derivatives with decreased membranotoxic properties are studied.

1. INTRODUCTION

In water system there is a hydration cage around each object (molecule) that can be realized as 2D space related to the 3D space of the solution interior, so water molecules in hydration layer have lower number of degrees of freedom, i.e., entropy falls. If solute is amphiphile, molecule has two different molecular regions in sense of hydrophobicity. In hydrophilic region, amphiphile molecules have polar groups that can form hydrogen bonds with water molecules from hydratation cage. In hydrogen bonding thermal energy is released, and scattering around gives positive entropic contribution so water molecules in hydratation layer on hydrophilic side of amphiphile are thermodynamically stabilized (SWM – stabilized water molecules) related to water molecules on hydrophobic side of a amphiphile molecule (NSWM non stabilised water molecules) [1-6]. With increasing amphiphile concentration in water, solution system entropy declines more and more so, on certain range of concentrations amphiphiles associate in aggregates (if amphiphile is detergent they form micelles on critical micelle concentration-CMC) over their hydrophobic sides (surfaces)- hydrophobic interaction, while NSWM leave to solution interior which results in increasment of system entropy [6, 7].

Formation of bile acid salt micelles, i.e., mixed micelles of phospholipids and bile acid salts as well as incorporation of bile acid anion monomers in lipid membrane are processes mainly determined by hydrophobic interactions. If some surfactant is more hydrophobic, it has a greater tendency for formation of micelles as well as greater membranolitic ability [8, 9]. Thus, it is important to know architecture of molecules and how hydrophobic surface depends on the structure of the molecule. Some molecules can have polar group that can be sterically sheltered with hydrophobic parts of the same molecule [10].

2. BILE ACIDS STRUCTURE: ANATOMY OF STEROID SKELETON

Bile acids are molecules with the skeleton of cyclopentanoperhydro-fenantrene, i.e., steroid compounds with mainly 24 carbon atoms. Bile acids enzimatically produced in liver of humans and other vertebrates are primary bile acids (cholic (C) and chenodeoxycholic acid (CD)). From them, after bacteriological transformation in the intestinal flora of the colon, secondary bile acids are obtained (deoxycholic acid (D), hyodeoxycholic acid (HD) and lithocholic acid (L))(Figure 1).

primary $\begin{cases}\text{cholic acid (C): } R_1\text{=OH, } R_2\text{=H, } R_3\text{=OH, } R_4\text{=OH} \\ \text{chenodeoxycholic acid (CD): } R_1\text{=OH, } R_2\text{=H, } R_3\text{=OH, } R_4\text{=H}\end{cases}$

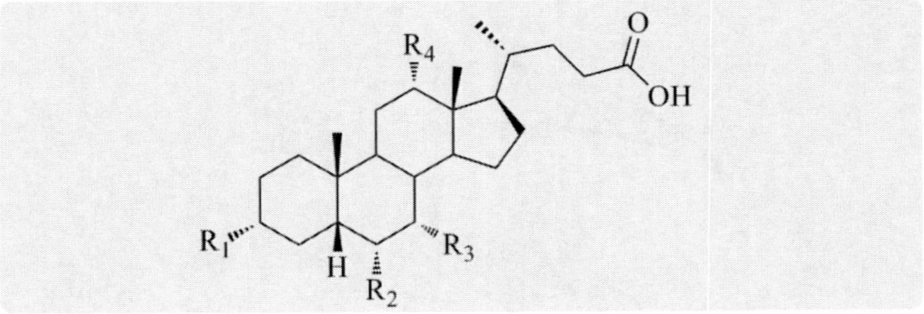

secondary $\begin{cases}\text{deoxycholic acid (D): } R_1\text{=OH, } R_2\text{=H, } R_3\text{=H, } R_4\text{=OH} \\ \text{hyodeoxycholic acid (HD): } R_1\text{=OH, } R_2\text{=OH, } R_3\text{=H, } R_4\text{=H} \\ \text{lithocholic acid (L): } R_1\text{=OH, } R_2\text{=H, } R_3\text{=H, } R_4\text{=H}\end{cases}$

Figure 1. Primary and secondary bile acids.

Primary and secondary micelles are hydroxy derivatives of 5β-cholanoic acid (Figure 2) [11-14].

In 5β-cholanoic acid hydrogens with axial bonds (bonds that are parallel to C_3 symmetry axis of cyclohexane) on convex surface of steroid skeleton represent β side of the molecule (β-hydrogens). Border area of van der Waals surfaces of axial hydrogens from β side of steroid system rings form convex surface of the molecule, while axial hydrogens on concave surface form α side of the molecule, α-hydrogens (Figure 3).

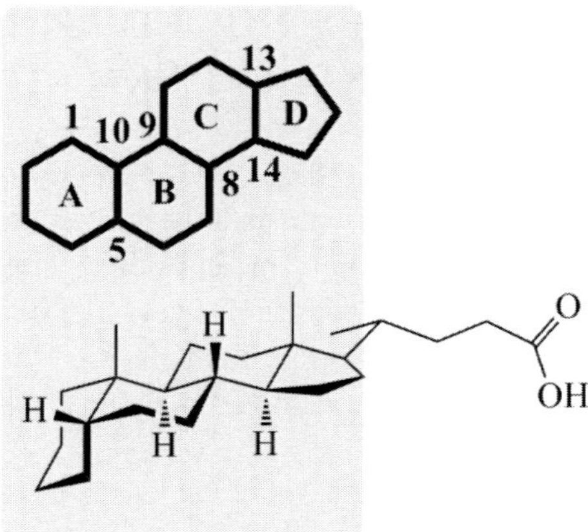

Figure 2. Conformation of 5β-cholanoic acid (CH), mutual binding of cyclohexane rings with cyclopentane ring of the steroid skeleton: A/B-*cis*, B/C-*trans*, C/D-*trans*.

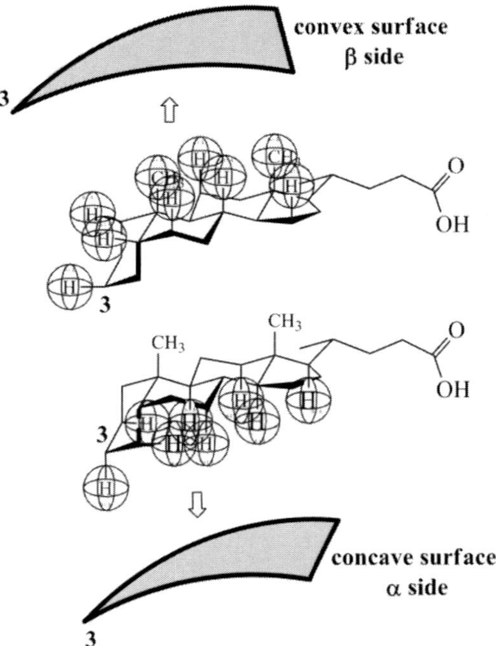

Figure 3. Geometric surfaces and steroid skeleton of 5β-cholanoic acid.

Border area of van der Waals volume of hydrogen atoms with equatorial bonds of appropriate cyclohexane rings of steroid skeleton of 5β-cholanoic acid form lateral side of a molecule, i.e., surface in the space between convex and concave plane. Equatorial hydrogens from lateral surface of steroid skeleton whose σ bonds form angle of +30° with steroid skeleton mean plane (SSMP) in a proper Newman projection formula (moving clockwise starting from mean plane) are also marked as α-hydrogen (i.e., σ bonds of these hydrogens related to σ bonds of α-axial hydrogen are switched for 60°). Equatorial hydrogens from lateral side of a molecule whose σ bonds in a proper Newman projection formula form angle of -30° with SSMP are also marked as β hydrogens (i.e., σ bonds of these hydrogen's are switched for 120° related to σ bonds of α-axial hydrogen)(Figure 4) [10, 14-16].

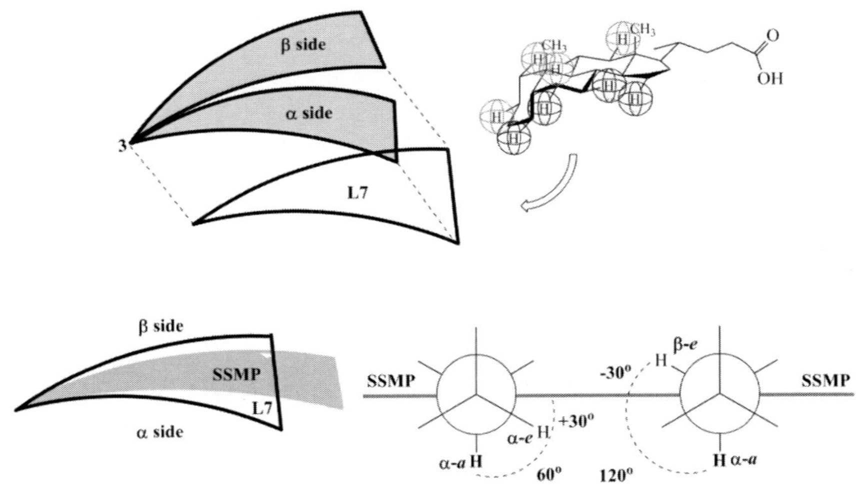

Figure 4. Geometrical surfaces and steroid skeleton of 5β-cholanoic acid: lateral side of a molecule.

If bile acid has α axial (a) hydroxyl group, water molecules from hydration layer can only be stabilized by hydrogen bonds from concave side of a steroid skeleton (Figure 5) [10, 14].

Bile acid with α equatorial OH group, which is, related to α axial OH group in Newman projection formula switched for 30° toward SSMP (i.e., it is on lateral side L7 of the steroid ring system), can stabilize water molecules from hydration layer from concave surface as well as from lateral surface (Figure 6). It can be concluded that α-(e)-OH more lowers whole hydrophobic surface of the steroid skeleton than α-(a)-OH group does [10, 14].

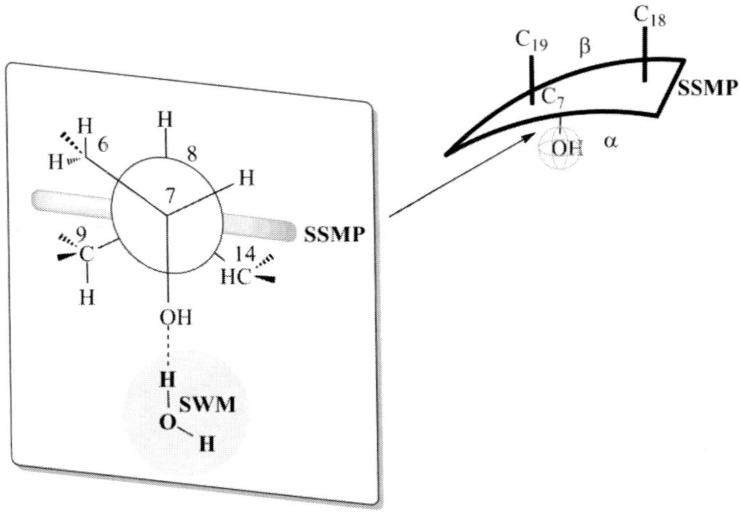

Figure 5. Newman projection of environment of C7-α-(*a*)-OH group of steroid skeleton, groups of steroid skeleton stabilizes water molecules (SWM) from hydration layer from concave side of a molecule.

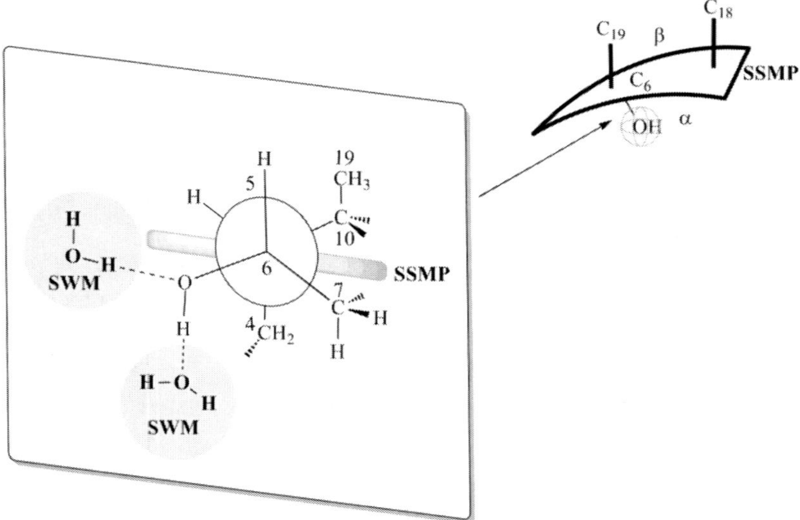

Figure 6. Newman projection of environment of C6-α-(*e*)-OH group of steroid skeleton that stabilizes water molecules (SWM) by hydrogen bonds from hydration layer from concave and lateral L7 surface of the molecule.

Molecule of bile acid with β equatorial hydroxyl group, which is in Newman projection formula switched for 120° toward SSMP related to α axial OH group, stabilizes water molecules from hydration layer from convex, i.e., lateral side of steroid skeleton by hydrogen bonds. Also, C7-β-(*e*)-OH group in greater extend lowers whole hydrophobic surface of molecule than α-(*a*)-OH or β-(*a*)-OH group does (Figure 7) [10, 14].

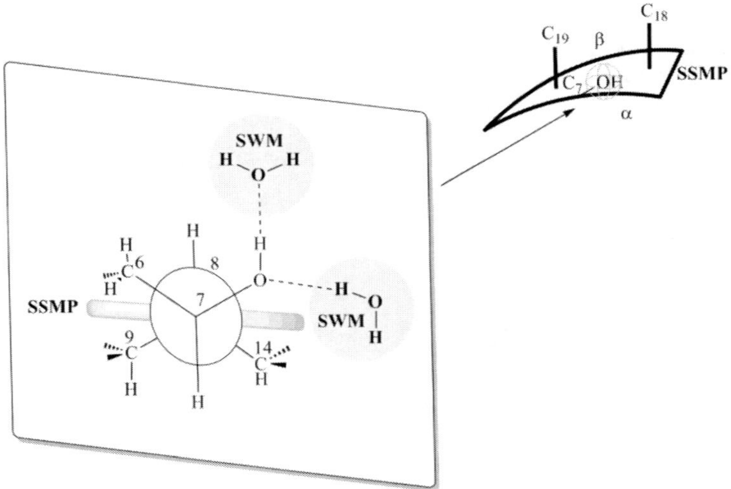

Figure 7. Newman projection formula of environment of C7-β-(*e*)-OH group of steroid skeleton that stabilizes water molecules (SWM) from hydration layer on convex and lateral L7 surface of the molecule by hydrogen bonds.

Experimentally, hydrophobicity of bile acid salts (molecules) can be expressed as logarithm of retention factor (capacity factor, log k) gained in reversed phase chromatography (RC) [17, 18]. In RC stationary phase represent hydrophobic surface so bile acid molecules adsorb over their biggest hydrophobic surface which is convex surface, i.e., β side of the steroid skeleton. During adsorption of bile acid molecules from their surface that is bounded for stationary phase molecules NSWM are released, Gibbs adsorption energy $\left(\Delta G_{ad}^{\circ} = RT \ln k + \underbrace{RT \ln \Phi}_{const.} \right)$ is proportional to whole change of entropy of hydrophobic interaction (Φ is parameter of chromatographic column, values ln k for different bile acids can be compared on the same chromatographic column). If chromatographic stationary phase is saturated with bile acid molecules, hydrophobic interactions between bile acid molecules are possible even over their lateral sides (Figure 8) [19].

Also, hydrophobicity of bile acids can be expressed with logarithm of partition coefficient, distribution of molecule between 1-octanole as lipid phase and water phase (log P). When bile acid molecule moves from water phase to lipid phase, whole amount of NSWM is liberated from hydration layer so log P is a measure for the whole hydrophobic surface of a bile acid (Figure 8) [20, 21]. Cholic and ursocholic acid have 3 hydroxyl groups in the steroid skeleton. However, ursocholic acid is C7 epimer of cholic acid. Thus, ursocholic acid in its B ring of steroid system of rings has β equatorial OH group, which, related to the cholic acid in hydratation layer significantly lowers number of NSWM, and by this, lowers values of hydrophobicity parameters of this molecule (Figure 8, Table 1). Chenodeoxycholic acid has only two OH groups in the steroid skeleton, so for CD hydrophobic surface appears also from α side of a molecule, i.e., from lateral L12 surface.

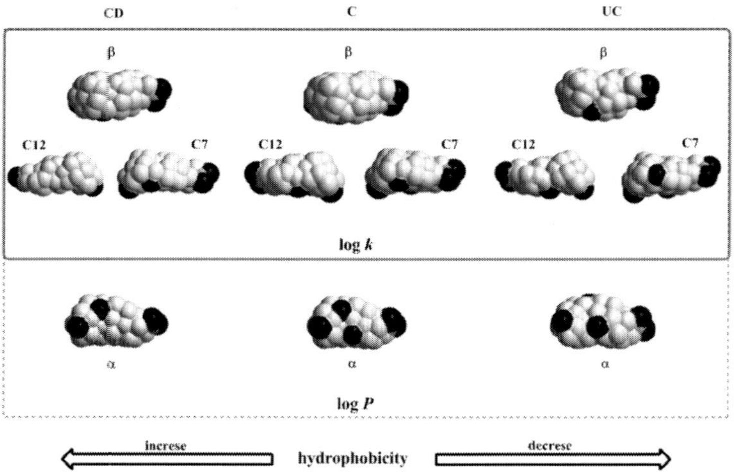

Figure 8. Log k determines hydrophobic surface from β and from lateral side of bile acid molecule, while log P determines whole hydrophobic surface (chenodeoxycholic acid (CD), cholic acid (C) and ursocholic acid (UC),

Table 1. Parameters of hydrophobicity [20]

	CD	C	UC
log P	3.28	2.02	0.92
log k	0.90	0.59	0

2. MICELLES OF BILE ACID SALTS AND THEIR MIXED MICELLES WITH PHOSPHOLIPIDS

According to the oldest, Smalls model, salts of cholic acid and their conjugated derivatives form primary micelles.

Two hydroxy derivatives of cholanoic acid also form primary micelles in water solutions if concentration of salt is low (up to 0,03 moldm^{-3} NaCl). Primary micelles have small dimensions, i.e., low aggregation number related to aggregation number of classic surfactant micelles (polar head- hydrophobic tail, for example sodium dodecilsulfat).

Aggregation number of primary micelles ranges from 2 (dimers) to 13,14 [11, 22-28].

According to structure, i.e., due to orientation of bile acid salt on border surface water-air it can be assumed that in interior of micelle, bile acid salts are associated by hydrophobic interactions of steroid skeleton (Figure 9). From aggregates of different sizes most stabile is dimer that is formed even when bile acid salt concentration is above critical micelle concentration [22].

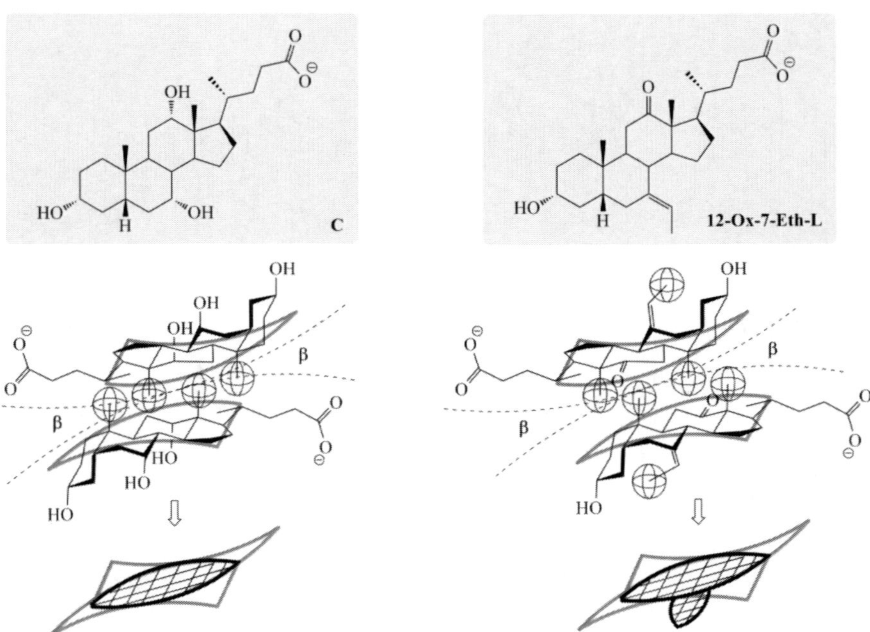

Figure 9. Primary micelles of bile salts.

In formation of cholic acid anion (C) binary micelle, due to convex surface of β side of steroid skeleton, not the whole β hydrophobic surface of C participates in association (Figure 9). Bile salt 12-oxo-7-etyliden-litocholat (12-Ox-7-Eth-L) has oxo group that has, due to it's α equatorial orientation, lower hydrophobic surface from convex side of the molecule, which improves aggregation of anions of 12-Ox-7-Eth-L (value of critical micelle concentration increases). However, derivative of 12-Ox-7-Eth-L has 7.8 mM value for CMC while C has CMC value 8.8 mM. This means that 12-Ox-7-Eth-L beside oxo group has higher tendency to micellisation than C. Bile salt 12-Ox-7-Eth-L has ethylidene group on the position C7, which is position where is minimum curvature of β side of steroid skeleton, i.e., where is the greatest overlap of convex surfaces of 12-Ox-7-Eth-L (Figure 9). This leads to increasing of entropic effect during formation of micelle of derivative 12-Ox-7-Eth-L due to higher number of NSWM that enter the interior of solution from the increased hydrophobic surface [29].

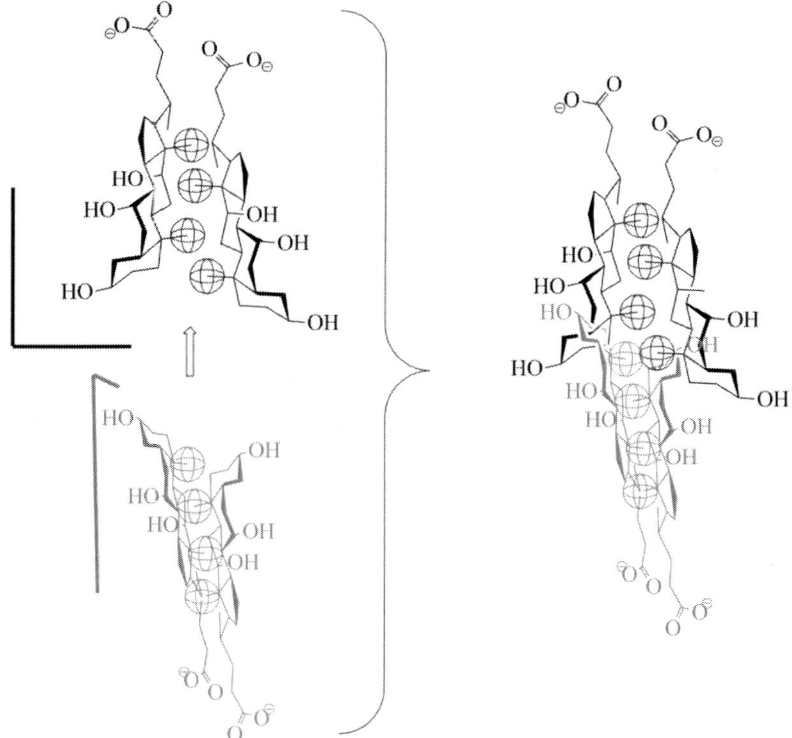

Figure 10. Primary micelles of cholic acid anion with aggregation number 4.

Presence of high concentration of NaCl in the solution of cholic acid anion causes formation of aggregates of about nine monomers. Influence of salt on increasing of aggregation number is explained in the following way:

- by lowering repulsive interaction between charged carboxyl groups of the side chain;
- partial dehydratation of nonionic hydroxyl group;
- salting out hydrocarbon part of a molecule.

Model of primary micelle composed of four cholate molecules is created by first forming the core from two molecules of bile salts (Figure 10), in which they are connected in a way that carboxylate groups of the side chain are positioned on the same size of the micelle. This core has longitudinal shape with two opposite sides; one with carboxylate groups and second, whose A rings of the steroid skeleton are *cis* connected. Such two cores connect (Figure 10) and form micelle with aggregation number four [30].

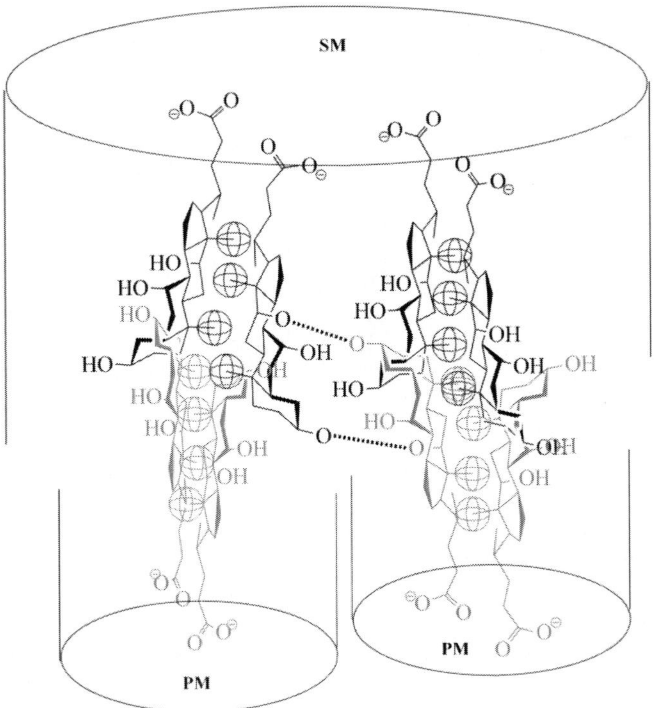

Figure 11. Secondary bile salt micelle.

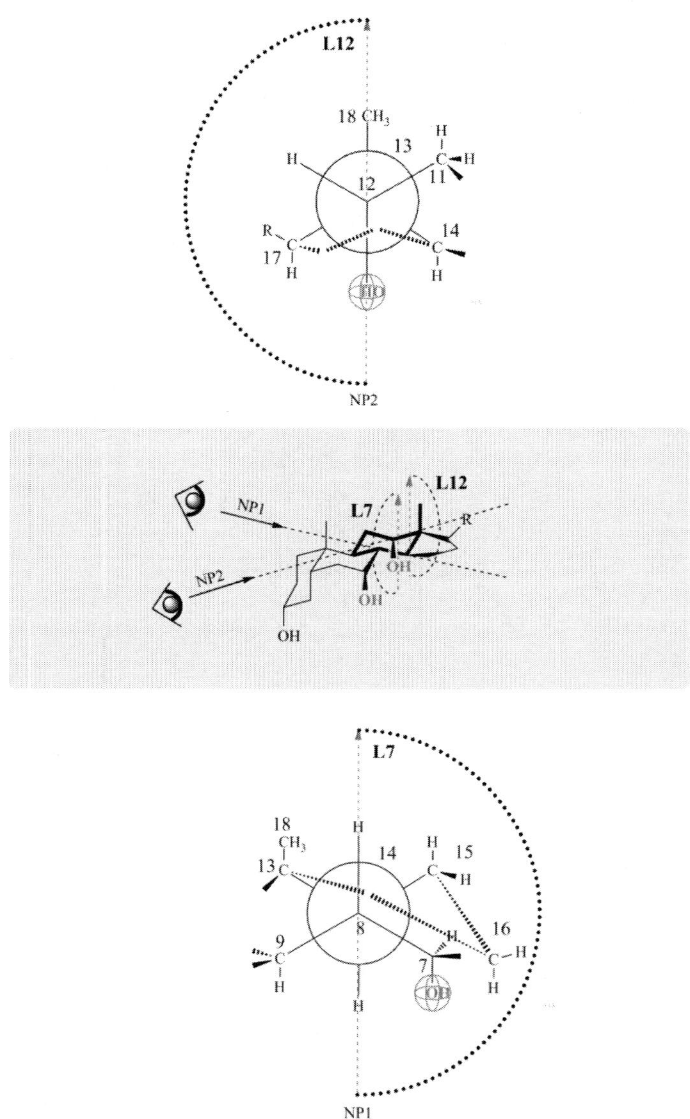

Figure 12. Steric environment of C7 and C12 axial OH groups of cholic acids.

From the standpoint of steric distribution it is possible to place up to ten monomers in the micelle, so molecules are bounded over their hydrophobic part and hydroxyl groups are oriented outward. Above this number each molecule enters in central space of the micelle, so part of the lipophile monomer is in contact with water and part of hydrophile part is in contact with other molecules in the micelle. Proof about binding of monomers over β-hydrophobic part of the steroid skeleton during micelle formation process is gained using NPR spectroscopy [22].

Secondary micelles are formed by association of primary micelles. In formation of primary micelles availability of hydrophobic surface of cholanoic acid anion derivative is lowered, and primary micelles mutually bind by hydrogen bonds (Figure 11). Increasing concentration of salts favors formation of secondary micelle, salting out effect of hydrohyl group happens and they mutually bind by hydrogen bonds [22, 25, 29-32].

There is a discussion in literature concerning presence and possibilities to prove forming of secondary micelles [25, 29-31]. According to equation:

$$\ln k = \underbrace{\frac{a-\bar{b}c}{\bar{\bar{b}}RT}}_{const.} - \underbrace{\frac{1}{\bar{b}}\ln\overline{\overline{CMC}}\,n}_{\tan\alpha}$$

for its hydrophobicity (ln k) bile acid anions belong to the common congeneric group and in the plane ln $k - n$ (aggregation number of micelle) they form linear congeneric group. This means that in formation of their micelles main attractive force is hydrophobic interaction between steroid skeletons. Bile acid anions (which, according to hydrophobicity form one common group) that not belong to line formed by objects of linear congeneric groups are outliners. For them next equation can be applied:

$$\ln k = \underbrace{\frac{a-\bar{b}c}{\bar{\bar{b}}RT}}_{const.} - \underbrace{\frac{1}{\bar{b}}\ln\overline{\overline{CMC}}\,n}_{\tan\alpha} + \frac{G^E}{bRT}\,.$$

In the previous equation there is excess Gibbs energy (G^E) in regard to Gibbs energy of hydrophobic interaction. Excess Gibbs energy probably comes from formation of hydrogen bonds between building units of bile salt micelles. Are hydrogen bond present between two identical hydrophobic (primary) micelles – i.e., in secondary micelles, or are they present in primary micelles (beside hydrophobic interactions) it cannot be concluded. Anions of bile acids that during the formation process have excess Gibbs energy, in regard to hydrophobic interaction, have next common elements: C3 α equatorial and C12 α axial (a) OH group. Due to steric hindering of C7 α axial (a) OH group with D ring of steroid skeleton in molecule of CD, presence of C7 α-(*a*)-OH group is not enough for formation of hydrogen bonds between building units of the micelle. Carbon, C7 with α-(*a*)-OH group in regard to C2 axis *subG* is in *cis* position related to atoms C15, C16 and C17 of the D ring of steroid skeleton, while C12 carbon with, as well α-(*a*)-OH group is in *trans* position [10]. *Cis* position of C7 atom (with group: α-(*a*)-OH) and D ring results in the proper Newman projection formula (Figure 12. NP1) C7-α-(*a*)-OH is in a position between synclinal (*sc*) and synperiplanar (*sp*) with C15 and C16 atoms of the D ring. This results in steric hindering of C7-α-(*a*)-OH group with D ring in L7 plane of the lateral side of steroid skeleton which makes harder process of hydrogen binding with building units from the same or different micelle, i.e., formation of secondary micelles. In Newman projection formula NP2 (Figure 12) C12 carbon atom (with group: α-(*a*)-OH) is in *sc* position in regard to C17 and C14 carbon atoms. However, other C atoms of the D ring are not localized in L12 plane of the lateral side of the steroid skeleton, so D ring sterically does not hinder observed C12-OH group [25, 29].

Kawamura proposed micelle model in the shape of disc, on the basis of studies of bile acid salt aggregates using spin labeled probe molecule [33]. In this model, micelles of hydrophobic surfaces of building units are oriented toward solution, and hydrophobic surfaces of monomers are oriented toward aggregate interior (Figure 13). Micelles in disc shape longitudinal axis of bile acid molecules are mutually parallel. This model of bile acid successfully explains low value of binding coefficient of the contra ion (cation) for the micelle surface in regard to spherical micelles of sodium- dodecylsulphate (sodium-laurylsulfat). Kawamuras model allows continual increase of the micelle size with the increase of equilibrium concentration of bile acid salts. This model is applied for micelles with small aggregation numbers usually for three hydroxy derivatives of bile acids, i.e., for big rigid micelles of two hydroxy derivatives of bile acids. In evolution of Kawamuras micelle probably first dimer aggregate is formed in type of Smalls micelle, which, in further development, instead of axial extended aggregates, forms micelle in the shape of disc. Importance of dimer aggregate in micellisation process is experimentally determined by Gouin and Zhu (NMR) [34]. They used bile acid molecules that are using spacers bounded in dimer shape. Application of dimer bile acids in mixture with monomer bile acids results in decrease of critical micelle concentration value, which implies to increased tendency to aggregate formation. Otherwise, common characteristic of Smalls and Kawamuras micelle is hydrophilic exterior and hydrophobic interior [14].

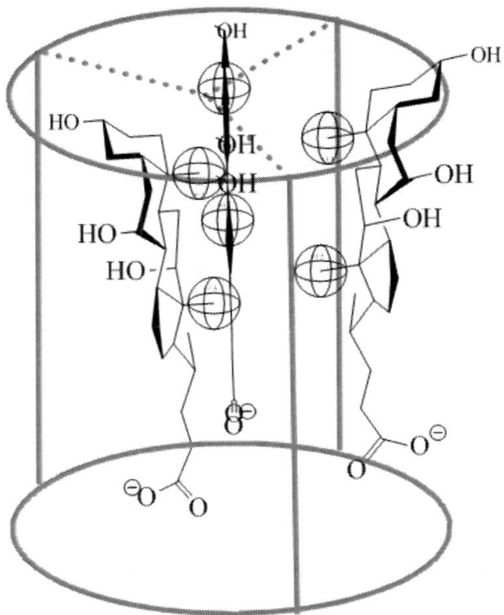

Figure 13. Kawamuras micelle of cholic acid anion model.

Global optimization and molecular dynamic simulation showed that sodium-cholate aggregate with 10 building units is the most stabile micelle comparing to lower aggregates of the same bile acid salt. In this aggregate there are 17 hydrogen bonds and one building unit surrounded by other sodium- cholate molecules. Such structure is extremely important since it shows that central particle can be replaced with a similar object, for example cholesterol or some steroid drug [35].

Oakenfull and Fisher measured specific conductivity of sodium-cholate and sodium deoxycholate and set model in which primary micelles of bile acids are formed by building hydrogen bonds between OH groups, while secondary micelles are formed by joining (hydrophobic interactions) over β sides of bile acid steroid skeleton (from primary micelles) [36-38]. This model is completely opposite from the most accepted Smalls model. However, Oakenfull and Fisher confirmed importance of hydrogen bond in formation of primary micelles on anions of dihydroxy derivatives of cholanoic acid. They noticed that sodium- hiodeoxycholate and sodium- ursodeoxycholate have lower tendency for micelle formation than sodium- deoxycholate, which cannot be explained by Smalls model, while their model explains different behavior of dihydroxy derivatives of cholanoic acid with higher stability of primary micelles (aggregates with hydrogen bonds). Hyodeoxycholic acid and ursodeoxycholic acid can form two types of primary micelles with hydrogen bonds: with open structure and with closed structure. Micelles with closed structure of ionized bile acids carboxylate group are 0.7nm apart, which leads to formation of repulsive forces so micelles are destabilized. Carboxylate group in micelle with the open structure are mutually sufficiently distant, but a large part of hydrophobic surface is in contact with water, which, from the aspect of entropy destabilizes micelle (aggregate). Deoxycholic acid forms micelle in which ionized carboxyle groups are maximum separated, and hydrophobic surface is less exposed to water. According to that, sodium-deoxycholate based on Oakenfull and Fisher model form more stabile micelle than sodium salts of hyodeoxycholic and ursodeoxycholic acid. Later, Vadrene et al. [39] measured the change of molar volume of bile acids and completely rejected Oakenfull and Fisher model of association over hydrogen bonds, preferring bile acid micelles that are formed by hydrophobic interactions (Smalls model).

Importance of Oakenfull-Fishers model is in that they did their measurements of conductivity in water solution of ethanol and other researchers did in water, so model of bile acid primary micelles with hydrogen bonds suggest existence of reversed micelles in hydrophobic environment, which is essential for promoter action of bile acids on transport of polar drugs through lipophilic barrier.

Among mixed micelles of bile acids with biomolecules, the most studied systems are with lecithin [22, 8]. Mixed micelles of cholate and henodeoxycholate have important role in solubilisation of cholesterol, bilirubin, etc. and have important application in biopharmacy [8].

The earliest model of mixed micelle of bile acid and lecithin was a disc model that was set in fifties and sixties of the last century.

Bile acid salts are proved to be great solubilisators of lecithin, since in average 1 mol of bile salt dissolve 2 mol of lecithin, while for classic aliphatic detergent it is necessary to have 20 mol of detergent for dissolving 1 mol of lecithin [22, 9]. Lecithin molecules have negligible small solubility, so it can be said that in micellar water solution dissolved lecithin in completely present in micellar phase. It is found that if in analyzed system molar fraction of lecithin is increased, number of lecithin molecule in mixed micelle increases from 2 to 80, and number of bile acid (salt) molecule increases from 12 to 52. It means that, with increasing of lecithin molar fraction, for solubilisation of one molecule of phospholipids the smaller amount of bile acid salt is necessary. According to Small, this phenomena can be best explained if we assume mixed micelle that is disc shaped (Figure 14) [22, 40-42].

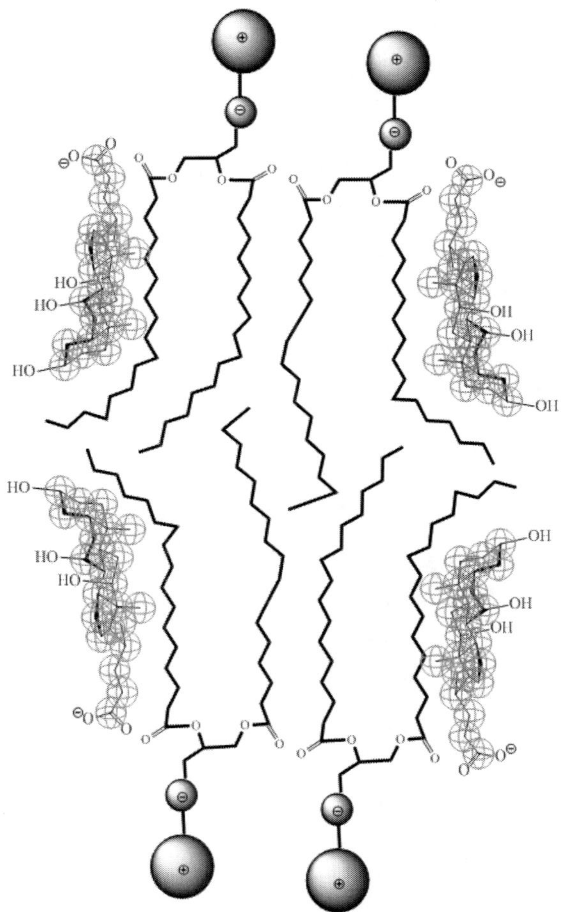

Figure 14. Historical Smalls model of mixed micelle of cholic acid anion and lecithin: disc shaped model.

In Smalls model lecithin molecules form two layers that are disc shaped (core of the mixed micelle) and whose ends are covered with hydrophilic phosphoryl-choline groups (from lecithin molecule), while on exterior surfaces there are hydrocarbon residues of fatty acids (from lecithin) for which bile acid salts are hydrophobically associated (in bile acid molecules β side of steroid skeleton is oriented toward hydrophobic surface of lecithin, while hydrophilic α side of steroid skeleton is facing water solution). According to Small model with increasing molar fraction of lecithin in mixed micelle, increasing of volume of hydrophobic micelle core (lecithin core) happens, and therefore increasing of cross sectional area of hydrophobic core. However, increasing of hydrophobic exterior surface (mantle of cylinder - disc) of the interior lecithin core with increasing of molar fraction of lecithin in mixed micelle is proportional to increasing of cross sectional area of lecithin core (πD_l) (Figure 15). Thus, the amount of bile acid salt molecule that is necessary for lecithin solubilisation with increasing its molar fraction in mixed micelle is proportional with increasing of circumference (πD_l) but not cross sectional area of lecithin core.

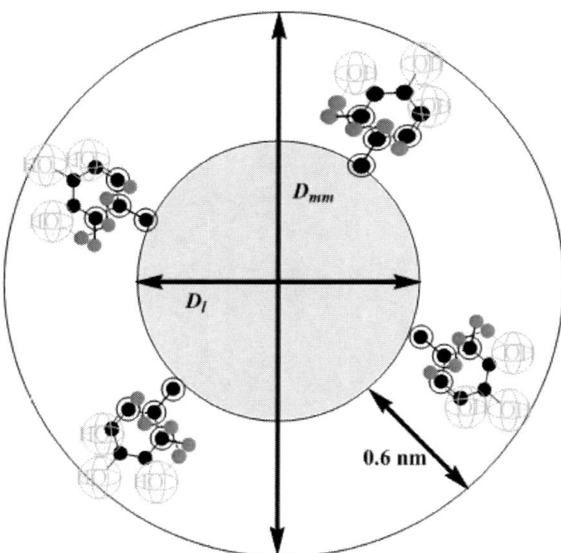

Figure 15. Cross section of mixed micelle normal to longitudinal axis of disc, D_{mm}, diameter of mixed micelle.

Using Smalls model it is theoretically possible to measure mass of mixed micelle using next approximations:

- bile acid molecules have elliptical cross section of the size 0.6 x 0.8nm;
- cross section surface of lecithin molecule in hydrophobic core of the micelles is 7 nm^2;

- disc height (mixed micelle) is gained taking into account that lecithin core is double layer;
- roughly, for each increasment of circumference of lecithin cross section core for 8 nm^2 it is necessary to incorporate, i.e., to add 2 molecules of bile acids (to each layer of double layer one molecule of bile acid.

Using previous approximations function of molecular mass of mixed micelle and molar fraction of lecithin/sodium cholate is calculated and it fits well to experimentally obtained curve of the same dependence, which supports Smalls disc model.

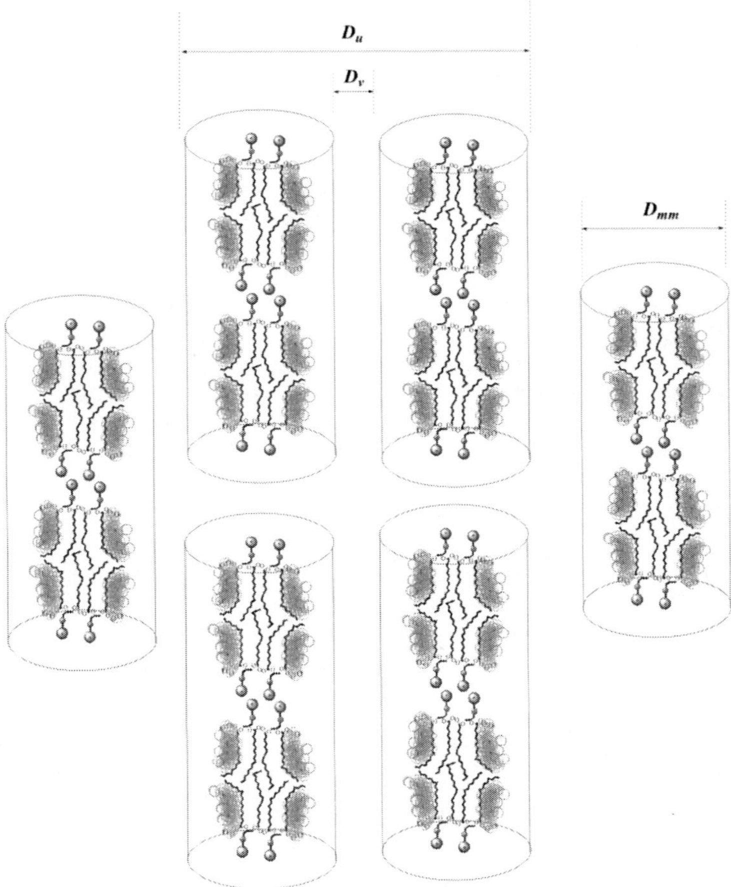

Figure 16. Hexagonal phase of lecithin and bile salt.

Further confirmations of disc model of mixed micelle were Smalls and Bourges examination of liquid crystal phase of sodium cholate and lecithin using X- ray diffraction [43]. Sodium- cholate and lecithin in presence of certain amount of water forms cylinders of undefined length packed in hexagonal crystallographic cell unit (along with the cylinder structure of disc shaped mixed micelle is repeated) (Figure 16).

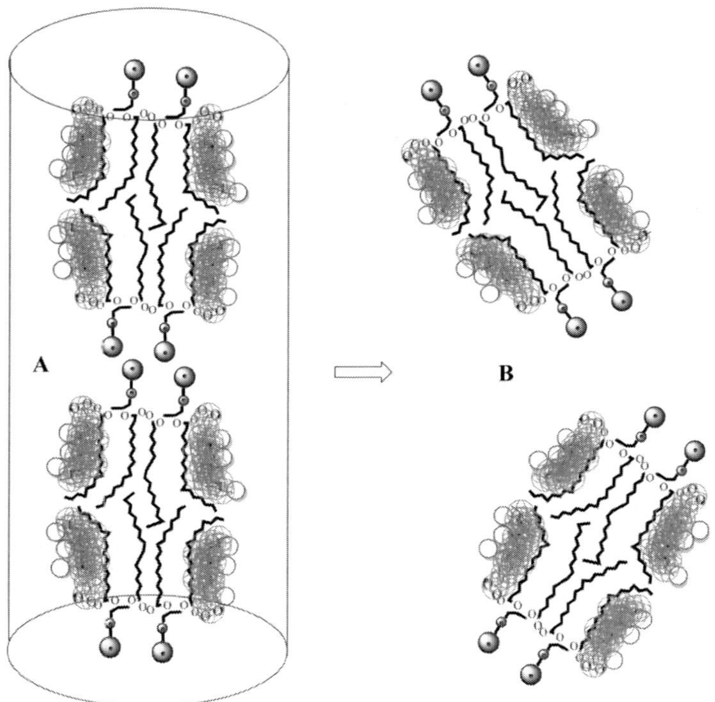

Figure 17. Phase transformation of hexagonal phase (A) into micellar phase (B).

By difractional experiment distances between middle of the cylinders is obtained (D_u). Distance D_u contains diameter of mixed micelle (D_{mm}) as width of water layer (D_v) placed between bile acid cylinder and lecithin. Small and Bourges determined D_u for different molar fractions of sodium cholate and lecithin at a phase transition of liquid crystals to micellar phase (Figure 17). They found linear dependence (line I) between experimentally gained D_u and molar ratio between bile acid salts and lecithin. Also, there is a linear dependence between calculated (according to Smalls model) cross section of mixed micelle (D_{mm}) and molar ration of building units (line II). Slopes of lines I and II don't differ, which confirms disc model of the mixed micelle. Differences in distances (D_v) from line I and II match widths of water layer between cylinders at phase transformations that is about 0.9 nm, i.e., water layer is about 3 water molecules thick. Thickness of water layer does not depend on molar ration of building units.

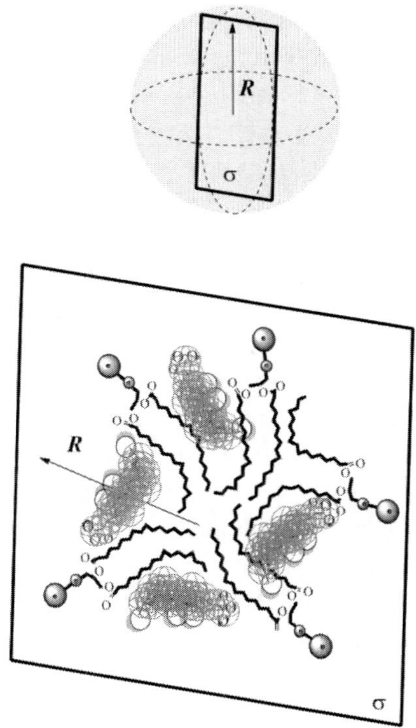

Figure 18. Radial model of mixed micelle of bile acid salt and lecithin in globular state.

For the shape of mixed micelle of bile acid salts and lecithin Shankland also suggested disc [44]. Today is the most expected radial model of the mixed micelle (Figure 18) according to which on high molar ration of bile salt/lecithin globular (more or less spheroid) mixed micelle is formed with radially placed lecithin molecules, and bile acid anions randomly located on the surface of mixed micelles between lecithin polar heads in a way that steroid skeleton is facing the inner hydrophobic phase (i.e., convex surface is normal to radius of mixed micelle) and concave hydrophilic surface of steroid skeleton is oriented to water phase [45-48]. Marrink and Mark used molecular dynamic simulations (MDS) and confirmed radial model of mixed micelles of sodium- cholate and lecithin. They found that C12 and C7 axial OH group of cholic acid are placed on the surface of the aggregate so they are hydrated or form hydrogen bonds with lecithin polar heads, while C3 equatorial OH group of cholic acid is little moved to interior hydrophobic phase of the micelle. Marrink and Mark did a MD simulation and examined a ternary system that included cholesterol. They found that incorporation of cholesterol in mixed micelle of sodium-cholate and lecithin do not disturb global structure of the aggregate, so cholesterol is also mainly radially oriented and cholesterols steroid skeleton in micellar pseudophase is solubilised with hydrocarbon lecithin segments, while C3 OH group is localized on the surface of the micelle [49]. With increase of lecithin bile acid sodium salt ratio, and increasment of systems water phase, radial globular mixed micelles extend into the shape of rod, i.e., in the shape of worm like mixed micelles with several turns in its length. Diameter of globular and worm like micelles is about 4 nm, which is twice as the length of the lecithin molecule [50].

According to Nichols and Ozarowski rod like mixed micelle of lecithin and bile acid anions on its longitudinal end has cap built from bile acid anions whose convex surface is parallel to aggregate radius: capped-rod mixed micelle model. In other parts of aggregates convex surface of steroid skeleton is normal to micelle radius [48]. Hausten et el. using Brownian derived dynamics (MDS) and coarse-grained model of sodium- cholate (C) and dipalmitoylphosphatidylecholine (DPPC) in experiment in which initial state was system consisted of lipid double layer of DPPC and monomer C. Phase transformation of lipid double layer happens saturated with C in worm like mixed micelle of DPPC and C. Starting from low concentration of C (but insufficient for solubilisation of lipid double layer) bile acid molecules incorporate in lipid phase of a double layer, so with gradual increase of C concentration pore formation happens in lipid double layer. On certain number of pores lipid bilayer with C enters phase transformation and becomes lipid bilayer-worm-like micelle [51].

4. INTERACTION OF BILE ACID SALTS AND PHOSPHOLIPIDS IN BIOLOGICAL SYSTEMS

Mutual interaction of bile acid salts and phospholipids were greatly studied when formation of bile and membranotoxicity of detergents were examined. Hepatocyte membrane from the side of bile canaliculus (canalicular or apical membrane) contains ATP-dependent transporters (exporters) for bile salts, primarily bile salt export pump, BSEP that moves bile acid anions from cytoplasm to canalicular lumen [52]. It is assumed that hepatocyte cytoplasm contains pool BSEP exporter and that cAMP, tauroursocholic acid and taurocholic acid stimulate incorporation of BSEP in hepatocyte epical membrane (it prevents that bile acid salt concentration exceeds critical micelle concentration and manifest membranotoxic effect in cytoplasm) [53, 54]. Lecithin, main bile phospholipids, from cytoplasm side of hepatocyte apical membrane using protein called multidrug resistance protein MDR3 (in humans MDR3, in mice protein Mdr2) translocate in canaliucular side of apical membrane. In environment of MDR3 protein canalicular side of the membrane is enriched in lecithin molecules [55]. In mices whose expression of protein MDR3 is genetically prevented, beside secretion of bile salts in bile, bile does not contain lecithin [55]. FXR (nuclear receptors: farnesoid X) activated by bile acids increases expression of MDR3 protein [56]. In cholesterol transport from hepatocyte to canaliculus probably MDR3 protein participates as well. In mices without Mdr2 flippase (transporter) bile does not contain cholesterol or contains it in a very small amount. However, infusion of bile salts in these mices increases secretion of cholesterol in bile, which suggests that micellar mechanism play role in secretion of cholesterol in bile [55](Figure 19).

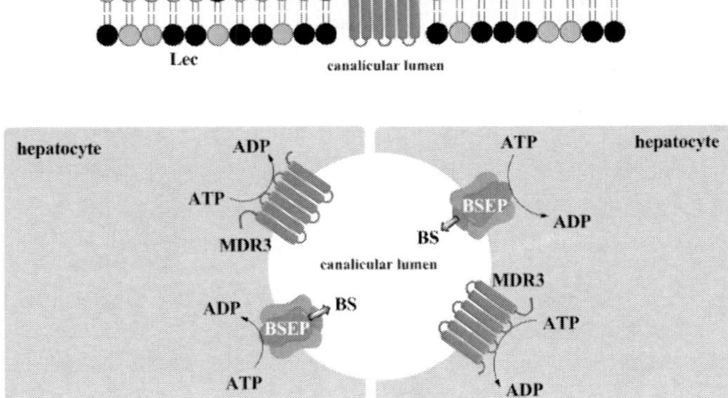

Figure 19. Main ABC transporters participating in secretion of bile salts and lecithin in canalicular lumen of the liver. Transversal diffusion (flip-flop) of lecithin from cytoplasmatic side of a hepatocyte membrane on canalicular side of the same membrane is a very slow process, so protein flippase MDR3 (BSEP = bile salt export pump, MDR3 = multidrug resistance protein 3).

For clarification of bile formation process it is necessary to examine ternary phase diagram of water, bile acid salt and lecithin in excess water, in regard to other components (Figure 20) [57, 58]. Each side of the triangle responds to binary mixture of corresponding components. Monophasic area (1ϕ) is isotropic water aqueous media in which micelles exist. Area 1ϕ below dashed line is a water solution of mixed micelles between bile acid salts and lecithin, and area above dashed line is water solution containing monomer micelles of bile acid anions and mixed micelles of bile acid anions and lecithin. Below the line of phase boundary 1ϕ (full line) there is a two phase area (2ϕ B) of water solution of mixed micelles and hexagonal phase (phase consisting of rod-like bile acid anion structure and lecithin in distribution similar to radial and worm like mixed micelles, wherein rods have hexagonal packing with water molecules between rod structures). Below this, two phase area there is a three phase system (3ϕ) of water solution of monomer bile acid anions on critical micelle concentration, hexagonal phase and lamellar liquid-crystalline phase. On the bottom of the clipping of a ternary phase diagram (Figure 20) there is again a two phase diagram (2ϕ A) of water solution of bile acid anion monomers below critical micelle concentration and lamellar liquid-crystalline phase.

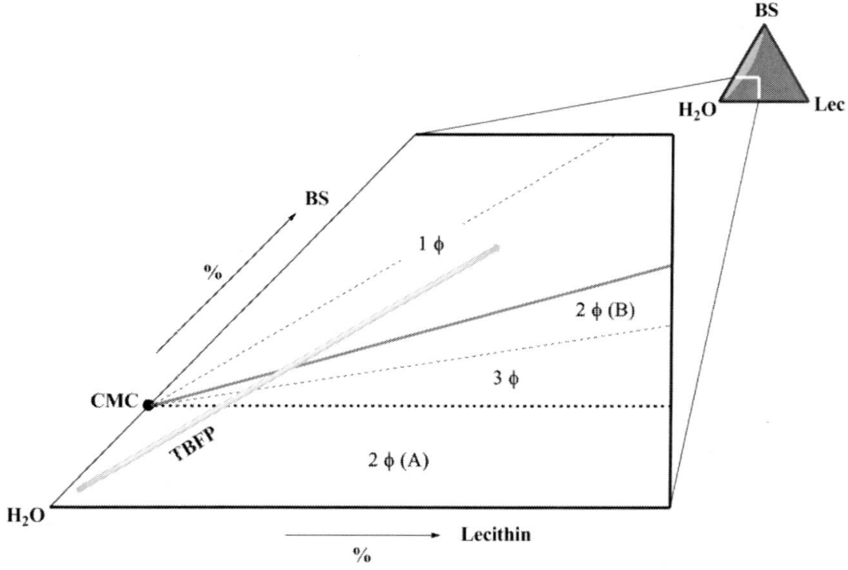

Figure 20. Ternary phase diagram, phase borders converge in point of critical micelle concentration (CMC) of analyzed bile acid (BS), TBFP = theoretical bile formation path.

Main event at bile formation in canaliculus theoretically can be identified if the line TBFR is followed in ternary phase diagram [58]. In gradual increase of canalicular concentration of bile acid anion monomer (area: 2φ A), monomers gradually implant in canalicular side of the hepatocyte membrane (this corresponds to lamellar phase) in a part where lecithin molecules form bud in a membrane. Bile acid anions destabilize membrane bud and unilamellar liquid-crystal vesicle are formed (UV) (that corresponds to lamellar phase) [59]. By using ultrafast cryofixation, Crawford et al. succeeded to visualize significant amount of unilamellar vesicle in lumen of canaliculus [60]. With further increasment of bile acid monomer concentration, monomer anions are subjected to flip flop process in UV so they are moved to the inner side of a membrane [61]. At saturation of UV with detergent monomers comes to crossings in three phase diagram since hexagonal phase is formed. With reapsorption of water, i.e., with concentrating of bile UV as lamellar-liquid phase completely disappears and again two phase system of water solution of bile acid anion mixed micelles and lecithin, i.e., hexagonal phase. Increasment of monomer concentration leads to formation of hexagonal phase so monophase water solution of mixed micelles is obtained. On higher concentration of lecithin worm like mixed micelles are formed and on higher concentration of detergent globular micelles are formed [58].

There is opinion on what in canaliculus unilamellar vesicles are not formed [62], only with gradual implantation of bile acid anions in apical membrane. Membrane destabilizes and new specific domains are formed. Monomers and bile acid micellar anions pull out lecithin molecules and form mixed micelles. This process does not correspond to ternary phase diagram because hepatocyte membrane would form hexagonal phase at the end of canaliculus (where the bile salt concentration is large enough that mixed micelles are formed) that would destabilize hepatocytes and probably cause their disintegration. Probably another, complex phase diagram corresponds to this process. Destabilization of canalicular side of hepatocyte membrane is probably of consequence of the way how bile acid steroid skeleton is incorporated. If steroid skeleton fits between lecithin polar heads with the convex surface facing lipid membrane phase, then below β side of the steroid ring system empty space is formed that should be filled with hydrocarbon segments of lecithin. However since lecithin has conformational mobile *sn*-1 palmotoyl residue related to unsaturated bile acid residues in *sn*-2 position, lecithin molecules should be specifically oriented toward bile acid anions, in a way that palmitoyl residue is adjacent to the empty space (that should be filled in), i.e., below bile acids convex side. This special orientation of lecithin molecule in membrane from canalicular side gives negative entropic change (configurational entropy), i.e., for conformational changes of hydrocarbon segment positive enthalpy change, so entry of steroid detergent in membrane results positive change in Gibbs energy of a lecithin membrane, i.e., lecithin molecules are thermodynamically destabilized.

They can leave a membrane and form mixed micelles even with monomer bile acid anions. Baskin and Frost found that sodium-taurodeoxycholate and sodium-cholate even on submicellar concentration form aggregates with 2-(6-(7-nitrobenzene-2-oxa-1,3-diazol-4-yl)amino)hexanoyl-1-hexadecanoyl-sn-glycero-3-phosphocholine in a way that steroid skeleton is in hydrophobic interaction with palmityne segment. One molecule of fluorescent- labeled phospholipid binds 2 molecules of sodium-taurodeoxycholate, i.e., sodium-cholate [63].

It was found that bromosulfophthalein (BSP) decreases lecithin secretion, i.e., of cholesterole and not affecting bile salts secretion [64]. Yamashita et al. showed that BSP form mixed micelle decreasing on that way their capacity to micellar solubilisation of lecithin and cholesterol [65]. This also supports the importance of bile salts in lecithin secretion.

It is known that sfingomyelin, with long saturated acyl segment (SM-S) does not enter bile although, beside lecithin, it represents main component of a hepatocyte apical membrane. However, bile contains traces of sfingomyelin with palmitine segment (SM-P) [66]. Selectivity in lecithin secretion regarded to SM-S can be explained in two ways.

First, SM-S forms more stabilized membrane with cholesterol due to more intensive secondary chemical bonds (induced dipol - induced dipole interactions) between long saturated hydrocarbon chains of SM-S and cholesterol steroid skeleton. They don't or hardly penetrate in stabilized bile acid anions membrane [67].

Palmitoyl segment of lecithin from antiperiplanar conformation (most favorable conformation for maximal interaction to cholesterol), is in vicinity of *sn*-2 unsaturated hydrocarbon chain, in *cis* configuration, and it should take a curled conformation in order to fill empty space around vicinal unsaturated chain which lowers interaction to cholesterol and bile acid anions can penetrate into the membrane.

Second, lecithin (Lec) forms thermodynamically more stabile mixed micelle with bile acid anions than with SM-S. Standard Gibbs energy of formation of binary mixed micelle and lecithin is $\left(\Delta G^{\ominus}_{mM} \right)$ [68]:

$$\frac{\Delta G^{\ominus}_{mM}}{RT} = \frac{\Delta G^{\ominus}_{M}(BS)}{RT} + \left(x^{mM}_{BS} \ln x^{mM}_{BS} + x^{mM}_{Lec} \ln x^{mM}_{Lec} \right) + \left(x^{mM}_{BS} \ln f^{mM}_{BS} + x^{mM}_{Lec} \ln f^{mM}_{Lec} \right) \quad (1),$$

where $\Delta G^{\ominus}_{M}(BS)$ corresponds to standard Gibbs energy of formation of monocomponent bile acid anion micelle, x^{mM}_{BS} and x^{mM}_{Lec} represent molar fractions of bile salt and lecithin in mixed binary micelle, and f^{mM}_{BS} and f^{mM}_{Lec} represent coefficients of activity of a building units in mixed micelle. Other term in equation (1) represents ideal Gibbs energy of mixing $\left(\Delta G^{\ominus}_{mix} \right)$ of monocomoponent micelle BS with pure lecithin phase, and it origins exclusively from configurational entropy of completely randomly distribution of different molecules in space- mixed micelle (i.e., entering of poorly soluble lecithin molecule from water phase in pseudo phase of a monocomponent micelle). Last term of expression (1) represent excess Gibbs energy $\left(G^{E} \right)$ because of deviation from ideal state. Excess Gibbs energy is:

$$G^{E} = H^{E} - TS^{E} \quad (2),$$

where H^{E} is excess enthalpy of formation real binary mixed micelle, while S^{E} corresponds to excess entropy of formation of mixed micelle between bile acid anion and lecithin. Standard Gibbs energy of formation of hypothetical binary mixed micelle of bile acid anion and SM-S is:

$$\frac{\Delta G^{\ominus}_{mM}}{RT} = \frac{\Delta G^{\ominus}_{M}(BS)}{RT} + \left(x^{mM}_{BS} \ln x^{mM}_{BS} + x^{mM}_{SM-S} \ln x^{mM}_{SM-S} \right) + \left(x^{mM}_{BS} \ln f^{mM}_{BS} + x^{mM}_{SM-S} \ln f^{mM}_{SM-S} \right)$$

First term in expressions for Gibbs energy of binary mixed micelles BS-Lec, i.e., BS-SM-S are identical, as well as the second term (Gibbs energy of mixing) at the same composition of mixed micelles (BS-Lec and BS-SM-S are formed in different systems). According to that, difference in thermo dynamical stability of binary mixed micelles BS-Lec and BS-SM-S is a consequence of different values of excess Gibbs energy. As lecithin and sfinglmyelin have the same phosphorylcholin group, in real binary mixed micelles BS-Lec and BS-SM-S there are identical synergistic interactions between positively charged nitrogen of phosphorylcholin group and carboxylate anion of bile acid- enthalpy effect. Thus, excess enthalpy is also nearly identical in this micellar system. However, excess entropy differs. In binary mixed micelles BS-Lec in lecithin molecule there is empty space (due to *cis* configuration of double bond) between *sn*-1 palmitoyl group and *sn*-2 unsaturated hydrogencarbon chain of appropriate acyl group in condition A (Figure 21) that allows conformational changes to palmitoyl saturated hydrogencarbon (depending on temperature). For mixed micelles BS-SM-S such conformational changes are not possible because all hydrogen carbons residues are saturated, i.e., empty space that initiate conformational changes is missing. With conformational changes of lecithin in mixed micelle BS-Lec, the volume of aggregate hydrophobic domain changes (change from state A to state B (Figure 21), so mixed micelles on certain constant temperature (T), pressure (p), i.e., number of building unit (N) can be observed as T,p,N ensemble (plenty of different micelles by volume and energy due to fluctuation on constant values of T,p,N). Excess entropy of such micelle is:

$$S^E = \frac{U^E - U_0}{T} + k \ln Q_{TPN} \tag{3},$$

where U^E represents excess internal energy of mixed micelle (on certain constant temperature), k = Boltzmann constant and Q_{TPN} is isothermal-isobar partition function. For mixed micelles BS-Lec and BS-SM-S approximation can be made that excess internal energies have the same value (similar energy synergistic interactions between different building units in both types of mixed micelles) so difference in thermodynamic stabilization between these two types of binary mixed micelles is reflected in difference of isotherm-isobar partition function:

$$Q_{TPN} = \sum_{\forall j} \sum_{\forall i} \exp\left(-\left(\frac{E_{ij} + pV_j}{kT}\right)\right) \tag{4}.$$

A summary in expression (4) refers to possible microstate of mixed micelle in which micelle reaches with fluctuating volume and energy, i.e., on conformational changes. As conformational changes in binary mixed micelle are more likely in BS-Lec than in binary mixed micelle BS-SM-S, binary mixed micelle BS-Lec occurs in greater number of microstates so more members in partition functions (4) corresponds to micelle BS-Lec.

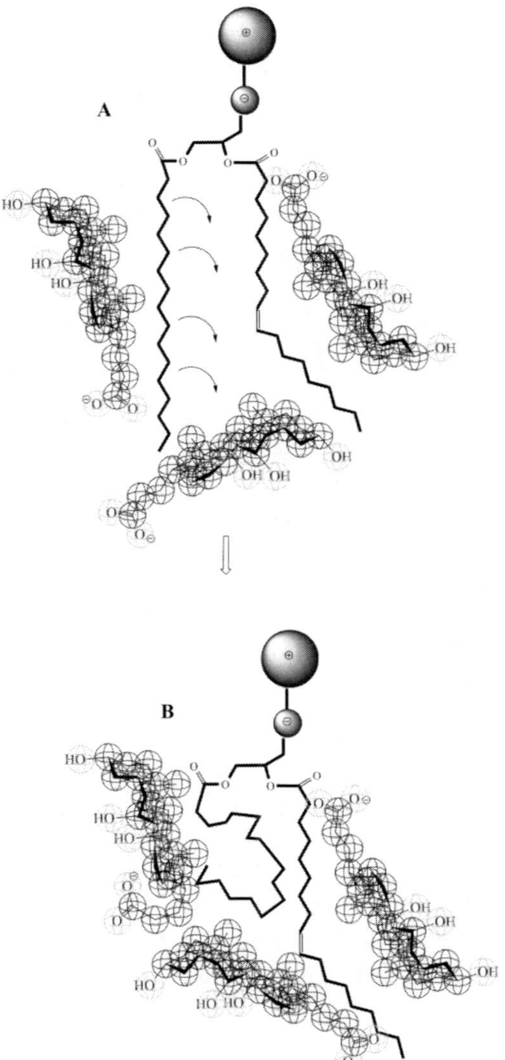

Figure 21. Empty space (condition A) in binary mixed micelle BS-Lec allows conformational changes, condition B corresponds to one micro condition of certain volume and energy on constant temperature, pressure and number of building units.

The system in relaxation tends to minimal value of Gibbs energy. In system (lumen of liver canaliculus) where formation of two types of mixed micelles is theoretically possible, i.e., BS-Lec and BS-SM-S, binary mixed micelles would be formed which results in greater decrease of Gibbs energy. As:

$$G^E = -kt \ln Q_{TPN} = -kt \ln \left[\sum_{\forall j} \sum_{\forall i} \exp\left(-\left(\frac{E_{ij} + pV_j}{kT} \right) \right) \right] \qquad (5),$$

excess Gibbs energy is more negative for binary mixed micelle BS-Lec, due to higher value of partition function, i.e., due to larger number of micro condition.

Table 2. Haemolytic potential of selected bile salt derivatives [9, 15]

Bile acids	CMC	Lys50	Lys100	G
	[mM]			
Deoxycholic acid	5.50	2.00	5.00	
Chenodeoxycholic acid	5.75	3.00	6.00	I
Cholic acid	8.00	4.50	8.00	
12-oxolitocholic acid	18.50	7.00	11.00	II
3,12-dioxo-5β-cholanoic acid	72.00	28.50	80.00	III
7-oxolitocholic acid	22.50	9.50	17.50	II
3,7-dioxo-5β-cholanoic acid	75.00	32.50	90.00	
12-oxochenodeoxycholic acid	65.00	35.00	70.00	III
7-oxodeoxycholic acid	60.00	25.00	60.00	
7,12-dioxolitocholic acid	100.00	58.00	120.00	
3,7-dioxo-12-α-hydroksi-5β-cholanoic a.	102.00	55.00	120.00	IV
Dehydrocholic acid	140.00	130	160<	V

Bile acid salts have long been used in experimental biochemistry for destruction of cell membrane. However, when bile acid salts are used as promoters of transport of some drugs through cell membrane as side effect membranotoxicity may occur [8]. In literature, toxic effects of bile acid anions are quantitatively expressed by hemolytic potential [69], that represents concentration of bile acid salt on which, *in vitro* experiment comes to 50% lyses of erythrocyte (Lys50), i.e., 100% lyses of erythrocyte (Lys100) [9]. There is correlation between critical micelle concentration value and hemolytic potential. Between CMC and bile acid salt concentration on which 50% of erythrocyte lyses happens (Lys50) Pearson correlation is 0.984 (p<0.01), while between CMC values and concentration of bile acid salts on which 100% of erythrocyte lyses happens (Lys100) Pearson correlation becomes significant and it is 0.994 (p<0.01) (Table 2). From hemolytic potential of examined bile acid salts it we can conclude that for deoxycholic, chenodeoxycholic and cholic acid 100% of erythrocyte lyses happens on their concentrations that are identical to their critical micelle concentration. Substitution of OH group with oxo group[‡] in examined bile acid anions decreases their hydrophobicity (number of equatorial oxygen atoms increases) so in keto derivatives 100% of erythrocyte lyses happens above their critical micelle concentration, and can be seen that hemolytic potential is particularly reduced for di- and three keto derivatives of cholic acid. Sodium salt of dehydrocholic acid on concentration of 160 mM does not reach maximum hemolytic potential.

Molecules with low CMC values have great hydrophobic surfaces, i.e., great power for solubilisation of lecithin, so building mixed micelles with lecithin from cell membrane disrupts membrane integrity.

In the plane of CMC and hemolytic potential, examined bile salts form five groups (Figure 23. and Table 2. G).

Each group has the following characteristics of the oxygen atom position (O) from hydroxyl and oxo group:

[‡] Introduction of the exocyclic double bond does not substantially change chair conformation of cyclohexane. Exocyclic double bond is in the same plane as equatorial substituent, which results in $A^{1,3}$ strain, therefore exocyclic double bond have equatorial orientation. Oxidation of α axial(α-a) OH groups of bile acids results in oxo group which by the corresponding Newman projection formula has an equatorial α (α-e) position (orientation). However, oxidation of (α-e) OH group (C 6OHgroups of hyodeoxycholic acid and hyocholic acid) results in oxo group with β equatorial orientation. Therefore, oxo group in cyclohexanon-like system have equatorial orientation, and α or β orientaion depends on orientaion of starting OH group. Position of oxo group in Newman projection is shifted for 60° relative to position of starting OH group[19,70].

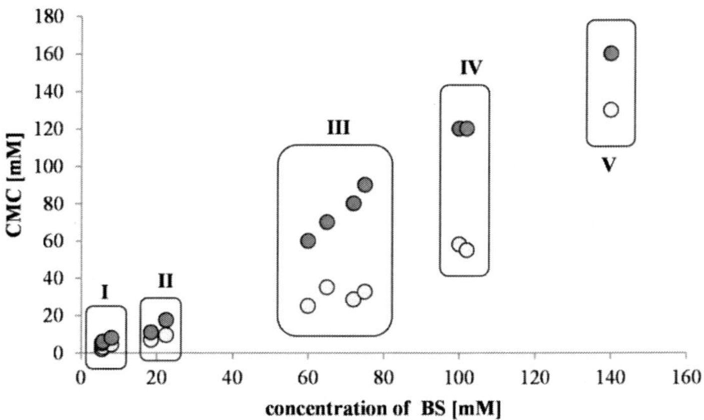

Figure 22. Grouping of bile acid salts in plane of critical micelle concentration and hemolytic potential: full circles = Lys50, empty circles: Lys100.

Group I = $1:\alpha(e)-O \wedge 1:\alpha(a)-O \vee 2:\alpha(a)-O$

Group II = $2:\alpha(e)-O$

Group III = $\left(1:\alpha(e)-O \wedge 1:\beta(e)-O\right) \vee \left(2:\alpha(e)-O \wedge 1:\alpha(a)-O\right)$

Group IV = $3:\alpha(e)-O \vee \left(1:\beta(e)-O \wedge 1:\alpha(e)-O \wedge 1:\alpha(a)-O\right)$

Group V = $1:\beta(e)-O \wedge 2:\alpha(e)-O$.

As it can be seen, groups are defined by the change in number of equatorial oxygen atoms, i.e., number of equatorial O atoms that control hydrophobic molecule surface. Equatorial O atoms stabilize water molecules from hydration cage from lateral side of steroid skeleton, i.e., from convex or concave side of a molecule depending on whether they have α or β orientation.

CONCLUSION

Hydrophobicity of bile acid salts is parameter that controls interaction between bile acid anions and phospholipids molecules, and manifests in bile formation as membranotoxic effect of detergent. By synthesis of fluorescent bile acid molecules, i.e., lecithin, and by using liver tissue with formed canaliculus with appropriate nano detectors (that can be introduced into the lumen of canaliculus) changes in the size of vesicles- micelles in bile formation can be followed.

REFERENCES

[1]   Kyte, J. The basis of the hydrophobic effect. Biophysical *Chemistry,* 2003, 100, 193-203.

[2]   Tanford, C. The hydrophobic effect and the organization of living matter. *Science,* 1978, 200, 1012-10118.

[3]   Chandler, D. Interfaces and the driving force of hydrophobic assembly. *Nature,* 2005, 437, 640-647.

[4]   Silverstein, T.P. The real reason why oil and water don' t mix. *J. Chem. Educ.,* 1998, 75, 116-118.

[5]   Haselmeier, R.; Holz; M.; Marbach, W.; Weingärtner H. Water dynamics near a dissolved noble gas. First direct experimental evidence for a retardation effect. *J. Phys. Chem.,* 1995, 99, 2243-2246.

[6]   Poša, M.; Kevrešan, S.; Mikov, M.; Ćirin-Novta, V.; Kuhajda, K. Critical micellar concentrations of keto derivatives of selected bile acids: Thermodynamic functions of micelle formation. *Colloids Surf. Biointerfaces,* 2008, 64, 151-161.

[7]   Poša,M.; Pilipović, A.; Lalić, M. The influence of NaCl on hydrophobicity of selected, pharmacologically active bile acids expressed with chromatographic retention index and critical micellar concentration. *Colloids Surf. Biointerfaces,* 2010, 81, 336-343.

[8]   Garidel, P.; Hildebrand, A.; Knauf, K.; Blume, A. Membranolytic activity of bile salts: influence of biological membrane properities and composition. *Molecules,* 2007, 12(10), 2292-2326.

[9]   Poša, M.; Kuhajda, K. Hydrophobicity and haemolytic potential of oxo derivatives of cholic, deoxycholic and cchenodeoxycholic acids. *Steroids,* 2010, 75(6), 424-431.

[10] Poša, M. Heuman indices of hydrophobicity in bile acids and compared with new developed and conventional molecular descriptors. *Biochimie,* 2014, 97, 28-38.

[11] Madenci, D.; Egelhaaf, U.S. Self-assembly in aqueous bile salt solutions. *Curr. Opin. Colloid Interface Sci.,* 2010, 15, 109-115.

[12] Hofmann, A.F.; Roda, A. Physicochemical properities of bile acids and their relationship to biological properties: an overview of the problem. *J. Lipid Res.,* 1984, 25, 1477-1489.

[13] Calabresi, M.; Andreozzi, P.; La Mesa, C. Supra-molecular association and polymorphic behaviour in systems containing bile acid salts. *Molecules,*2007, 12(8), 1731-1754.

[14] Poša, M. Hydrophobicity and self-association of bile acids with a special emphasis on oxo derivatives of 5-β-cholanic acid. *Current OrganicChemistry,* 2012, 16(16), 1876-1904.

[15] Poša, M. QSPR study of the effect of steroidal hydroxy and oxo substituents on the critical micellar concentrations of bile acids. *Steroids,* 2011, 76(1-2), 85-93.

[16] Poša, M.; Farkaš, Z. Cholesterol solubilization by oxo derivatives of selected bile acids and their osmotic resistance. *Collect. Czech. Chem. Commun.,*2010, 75(8), 767-784.

[17] Natalini, B.; Sardella, R.; Camaioni, E.; Gioiello, A.; Pellicciari, R. Correlation between CMC and chromatographic index: simple and effective evaluation of the hydrophobic/hydrophilic balance of bile acids. *Anal. Bioanal. Chem.,* 2007, 388, 1681-1688.

[18] Natalini, B.; Sardella, R.; Camaioni, E.;Macchiarulo, A.; Gioiello, A.; Carbone, G.; Pellicciari, R. Derived chromatographic indices as effective tools to study the self-aggregation process of bile acids. *J. Pharm. Biomed. Anal.,* 2009, 50, 613-621.

[19] Poša, M.; Bjedov, S.; Sebenji, A.; Sakač, M. Wittig reaction (with ethylidene triphenylphosphorane) of oxo-hydroxy derivatives of 5β–cholanic acid: hydrophobicity and haemolytic potential of derived ethylidene derivatives. *Steroids,*2014, 86, 16-25.

[20] Roda, A.; Minutello, A.; Angellotti, M.A.; Fini. A. Bile acid structure-activity relationships: evaluation of bile acids lipophilicity using 1-octanol/water partition coefficient and reverse phase HPLC. *J. LipidRes.,* 1990, 31, 1433-1443.

[21] Lucangioli, S.E.; Carducci, C.N.; Tripodi, V.P.; Kenndler, E. Retention of bile salts in micellar electrokinetic chromatography: relation of capacity factor to octanol–water partition coefficient and critical micellar concentration. *J. Chromatogr. B,* 2001, 765, 113–120.

[22] Small, D.M. In: The bile acids; Nair, P.P.; Kritchevsky, D.; Eds.; Plenum Press: New York, 1977; Vol. 1, pp. 249-356.

[23] Kratohvil, J.P.; Hsu, W.P.; Kwok, D.I. How large are the micelles of di-a-hydroxy bile salts at the critical micellization concentrations in aqueous electrolyte solutions? Results from sodium taurodeoxycholate and sodium deoxycholate. *Langmir,* 1986, 2, 256-258.

[24] Funasaki, N.; Nomura, M.; Ishikawa, S.; Neya, S. Hydrophobic self-association of sodium taurochenodeoxycholate and tauroursodeoxycholate. *J. Phys. Chem. B,* 2000, 104, 7745-7751.

[25] Poša, M.; Sebenji, A. Determination of the number avarage aggregation numbers of bile salt micelles with a special emphasis on their oxo derivatives – the effect of the steroid skeleton. *Biochim. Biophys. Acta – Gen. Sub.,* 2014, 1840 1072-1082.

[26] Sugioka, H.; Matsuoka, K.; Moroi, Y. Temperature effect on formation of sodium cholate micelles. *J. Colloid Interface Sci.,* 2003, 259, 156-162.

[27] Ninomiya, R.; Matsuoka, K.; Moroi, Y. Micelle formation of sodium chenodeoxycholate and solubilization into the micelles: comparison with other unconjugated bile salts. *Biochim. Biophys. Acta,* 2003, 1634, 116-125.

[28] Coello, A.; Meijide, F.; Rodríguez Núñez, E.; Vázquez Tato, J. Aggregation behavior of bile salts in aqueous solution. *J. Pharm. Sci.,* 1996, 85(1), 9-15.

[29] Poša, M.; Bjedov, S.; Škorić, D.; Sakač, M. Micellization parameters (number average aggregation number and critical micellar concentration)of bile salt 3 and 7 ethylidene derivatives: role of the steroidal skeleton II. *Biochim. Biophys. Acta – Gen. Sub.,* 2015, 1850, 1345-1353.

[30] Poša, M.; Guzsvány, V.; Csanádi, J.; Borbás, J.; Gaál, F. Study of Assotiation of 12-Monoketocholic Acid by ^{1}H NMR Relaxation *Method. Acta Chim. Slov.,* 2009, 56(4), 807-814.

[31] Pártai, L.B.; Jedlovszky, P.; Sega, M. Molecular aggregates in aqueous solutions of bile acid salts. Molecular dynamics simulation study. *J. Phys. Chem. B,* 2007, 111, 9886-9896.

[32] Pártai, L.B.; Sega, M.; Jedlovszky, P. Counterion binding in the aqueous solutions of bile acid salts, as studied by computer simulation methods. *Langmuir,* 2008, 24, 10729-10736.

[33] Kawamura, H.; Murata, Y.; Yamaguchi, T.; Igimi, H.; Tanaka, M.; Sugihara, G.; Kratohvil, J.P. Spin-label studies of bile salt micelles. *J. Phys. Chem.,* 1989, 93, 3321-3326.

[34] Gouin, S.; Zhu, X.X. Fluorescence and NMR studies of the effect of a bile acid dimer on the micellization of bile salts. *Langmuir,* 1998, 14, 4025-4029.

[35] Jójárt, B.; Viskolc, B.; Poša, M.; Fejer, Sz. Global optimization of cholic acid aggregates. *The Journal of Chemical Physics*, 2014, 140, 1443021-1443027.

[36] Oakenfull, D.G.; Fisher, L.R. The role of hydrogen bonding in the formation of bile salt micelles. *J. Phys. Chem.*, 1977, 81, 1838-1841.

[37] Oakenfull, D.G.; Fisher, L.R. Reply to "Comments on the role of hydrogen bonding in the formation of bile salt micelles." *J. Phys. Chem.*, 1978, 82, 2443-2445.

[38] Fisher, L.R.; Oakenfull, D.G. The role of hydrogen bonding in the formation of bile salt micelles. 2. A demonstration of geometric effects on the stabilizing role of hydrogen bonding *J. Phys. Chem.*, 1980, 84, 936-937.

[39] Vadnere, M.; Natarayan, R.; Lindenbaum, S. Apparent molal volumes of bile salts in water and water-d solution. *J. Phys. Chem.*, 1980, 84(15), 1900-1903.

[40] Small, D.M. Physicochemical studies of cholesterol gallstone formation. *Gastroenterology*, 1967, 52, 607-610.

[41] Small, D.M; Bourges, M. Lyotropic paracrystalline phases obtained with ternary and quaternary systems of amphiphilic substances in water: Studies on aqueous systems of lecithin, bile salt, and cholesterol.. *M. Mol. Crystals*, 1966, 1, 544-561.

[42] Bourges, M.; Small, D. M.; Dervichian, D. G. Biophysics of lipid associations. III. Quaternary systems lecithin-bile salt-cholesterol-water. *Biochim. Biophys. Acta, Lip. Lipid Metabol.* 1967, 144, 189-201.

[43] Small, D.M.; Penkett, S.A.; Chapman, D. Studies on simple and mixed bile salt micelles by nuclear magnetic resonance spectroscopy. *Biochem. Biophys. Acta*, 1969, 176, 178-189.

[44] Shankland, W. The equilibrium and structure of lecithin-cholate mixed micelles. *Chem. Phys. Lipids,* 1970, 4, 109-130.

[45] Ulmius, J.; Lindblom, G.; Wennerström, H.; Johansson, L. B.; Fontell, K.; Söderman, O.; Arvidson, G. Molecular organization in the liquid-crystalline phases of lecithin-sodium cholatewater systems studied by nuclear magnetic resonance. *Biochemistry,* 1982, 21, 1553-1560.

[46] Hjelm, R. P.; Thiyagaragan, P.; Sivia, D. S.; Lindner, P.; Alkan, H.; Schwahn, D. Small-angleneutron scattering from aqueous mixed colloids of lecithin and bile salt. *Progr. Colloid. Polym. Sci.*, 1990, 81, 225–231.

[47] Hjelm, R. P.; Schteingart, C. D.; Hofmann, A. F.; Thiyagarajan, P. Structure of Conjugated Bile Salt-Fatty Acid-Monoglyceride Mixed

Colloids: Studies by Small-Angle Neutron Scattering. *J. Phys. Chem. B,* 2000, 104, 197-211.

[48]   Nichols, J. W.; Ozarowski, J. Sizing lecithin-bile salt mixed micelles bysize-exclusion high-performance liquid chromatography. *Biochemistry,*1990, 29, 4600–4606.

[49]   Marrink, S. J.; Mark, A. E. Molecular dynamics simulations of mixed micelles modeling human bile. *Biochemistry,* 2002, 41, 5375-5382.

[50]   Cohen, D. E.; Thurston, G. M.; Chamberlin, R. A.; Benedek, G. E; Carey, M. E. Laser light scattering evidence for a common wormlike growth structure of mixed micelles in bile salt- and strain-chain detergentphosphatidylcholine aqueous systems: relevance to the micellar structure of bile. *Biochemistry,* 1998, 37, 14798–14814.

[51]   Haustein, M.; Schiller, P.; Wahab, M.; Mogel, H. J. Computer simulations of the formation of bile salt micelles and bile salt/DPPC mixed micelles in aqueous solutions. *J. Solution Chem.,* 2014, 43, 1755-1770.

[52]   Nishida, T.; Gatmaitan, Z.; Che, M. X.; Arias, I. M. Rat liver canalicularmembrane vesicles containingan ATP-dependent bile acid transport system. *Proc. Natl. Acad. Sci. USA,* 1991, 88, 6590–6594.

[53]   Kipp, H.; Pichetshote, N.; Arias, I. M. Transporters on demand: Intrahepatic pools of canalicular ATPbindingcassette transporters in rat liver. *J. Biol. Chem.,* 2001, 276, 7218–7224.

[54]   Stieger, B. The role of the sodium-taurocholate cotransporting polypeptide (NTCP) and of the bilesalt export pump (BSEP) in physiology and pathophysiology of bile formation. *Handb. Exp. Pharmacol.,* 2011, 201, 205–259.

[55]   Boyer, J. L. Bile formation and Sekretion. *Compr. Physiol.,* 2013, 3(3), 1035–1078.

[56]   Huang, L.; Zhao, A.; Lew, J. L.; Zhang,T.; Hrywna, Y.; Thompson, J. R.; de Pedro, N.; Royo, I.; Blevins, R. A.; Pelaez, F.; Wright, S. D.; Cui, J. Farnesoid X receptor activates transcription of the phospholipidpump MDR3. *J. Biol. Chem.,* 2003, 278, 51085–51090.

[57]   Small, D.M; Bourges, M.; Dervichian, D. G. Ternary and quaternary aqueous systems containing bile salts, lecithin and cholesterol. *Nature,* 1966, 211, 816-818.

[58]   Cohen, E. D.; Angelico, M.; Carey, M. C. Structural alterations in lecithin-cholesterol vesicles following interactions with monomeric and micellar bile salts: physical-chemical basis for subselection of biliary

lecithin species and aggregative states of biliary lipids during bile formation. *J. Lipid Res.*, 1990, 31, 55-70.

[59] Crawford, A. R.; Smith, A. J.; Hatch, V. C.; Oude, E. R.; Borst, P.; Crawford, J. M. Hepatic secretion ofphospholipid vesicles in the mouse critically depends on mdr2 or MDR3 P-glycoproteinexpression. Visualization by electron microscopy. *J. Clin. Invest.*, 1997, 100, 2562–2567.

[60] Crawford, J. M.; Mockel, G. M.; Craword, A. R.; Hagen, S. J.; Hatch, V. C.; Barnes, S.; Godleski, J. J.; Carey, M. C. Imaging biliary lipid secretion in the rat: ultrastructural evidence for vesiculation of the hepatocyte canalicular membrane. *J. Lipid Res.*, 1995, 36, 2147-2163.

[61] Cabral, D. J.; Small, D. M.; Lilly, H. S.; Hamilton, J. A. Transbilayer movement of bile acids inmodel membranes. *Biochemistry*1987, 26, 1801-1804.

[62] Oude, Elferink, R. P.J.; Tytgat, G. N. J.; Groen, A. K. The role of mdr2 P-glycoprotein in hepatobiliarylipid transport. *FASEB J.*, 1997, 11, 19–28.

[63] Baskin, R.; Frost, L. Bile salt-phospholipid aggregation at submicellar concentrations. Colloids Surf. Biointerfaces, 2008, 62(2), 238-242.

[64] Miura, H.; Tazuma, S.; Kajiyama, G. Partial characterization of regulation of biliary lecithin hydrophobicity: association with organic anion-induced solute cholestasis in rats. *Biochem. J.*, 1995, 312, 795-797.

[65] Yamashita, G.; Tazuma, S.; Kajiyama, G. Effects of organic anions on biliary lipid secretion in rats. Importance of association with biliary lipid structures. *Biochem. J.*, 1992, 286, 193-196.

[66] Nibbering, C. P.; Carey, M. C, Sphingomyelins of rat liver: biliary enrichment with molecular species containing 16:0 fatty acids as compared to canalicular-enriched plasma membranes. *J. Membr. Biol.*, 1999, 167, 165-171.

[67] Eckhard, E. R. M.; Moschetta, A.; Renooj, W.; Goerdayal, S. S.; van Berge-Henegouwen, G. P.; van Erpecum, K. J. Asymmetric distribution of phosphatidylcholine and sphingomyelin between micellar and vesicular phases: potential implications for canalicular bile formation. *J. Lipid. Res.*, 1999, 40, 2022-2033.

[68] Poša, M. Mixed micelles of binary surfactant mixtures: Tween 40 - Na-3,12-dioxo-5β-cholanoate; Tween 80 - Na-3,12-dioxo-5β-cholanoate and their thermodynamic description-characterization. *Chem. Eng. Res. andDes.*, 2014, 92(12), 1826-1839.

[69] Bowe, C.L.; Mokhtarzadeh, L.; Venkatesen, P.; Babu, S.; Axelrod, H.; Sofia, M.J.; Kakarla, R.; Chan, T.Y.; Kim, J.S.; Lee, H.J.; Amidon, G.L.; Choe, S.Y.; Walker, S.; Kahne, D. Desing of compounds that increase the absorption of polar molecules. *Proc. Natl. Acad. Sci. USA*, 1997, 94, 12218-12223.

[70] Poša, M.; Farkaš, Z. Cholesterol solubilization by oxo derivatives of selected bile acids and their osmotic resistance. *Collect. Czech. Chem. Commun.*, 2010, 75(8), 767-784.

In: Bile Acids
Editor: Aileen Murphy

ISBN: 978-1-63484-074-3
© 2016 Nova Science Publishers, Inc.

Chapter 3

BILE ASPIRATION: A HOST FACTOR MODULATING CHRONIC RESPIRATORY INFECTION

*Stephanie Flynn[1], David F. Woods[1],
Muireann Ní Chróinín[2], David Mullane[2],
Claire Adams[1], F. Jerry Reen[1] and Fergal O'Gara[1,3]*

[1]BIOMERIT Research Centre, Department of Microbiology,
University College Cork, Cork, Ireland
[2]Paediatric CF Clinic, Cork University Hospital, Cork, Ireland
[3]School of Biomedical Sciences, Curtin Health Innovation
Research Institue, Curtin University, Perth, Australia

ABSTRACT

Bile acid dysmetabolism has long been associated with a broad spectrum of diseases such as diabetes, gastrointestinal disease and obesity (Jones et al. 2014). More recently, however, the aspiration of bile acids into the lungs of respiratory patients has been implicated in the pathophysiology of chronic respiratory disease including cystic fibrosis (CF), chronic obstructive pulmonary disease (COPD) and asthma (Hallberg et al. 2004, Sweet et al. 2009, Mertens et al. 2011, Pauwels et al. 2012, Reen et al. 2012). Chronic respiratory infections are a leading cause of morbidity and mortality in these patients, particularly in the CF population. Once pathogens have transitioned from an acute to chronic biofilm lifestyle, antibiotic treatments become largely ineffective, severely limiting the clinical management of respiratory diseases. Whilst much is known about the molecular mechanism underpinning this lifestyle switch, little is known about the signals that trigger this detrimental behavioural change. Due to its immense clinical significance it is imperative to identify the signals and pathways responsible for this switch. These subsequently be targeted with novel therapeutic strategies.

It has been known for many years that gastro-oesophageal reflux (GOR) is prevalent in the CF population (Button et al. 2005, Blondeau et al. 2008a, Blondeau et al. 2010). Up to 80% of CF patients exhibit symptoms, with GOR positive patients exhibiting more severe lung disease. Recent evidence suggests that bile, which is refluxed during episodes of GOR, is aspirated into the lungs and is responsible for this observed pathology where it is estimated that aspiration could be as high as 80%. The effectiveness of surgical treatment known as a Nissen fundoplication in controlling progressive lung decline and the limitations of conventional therapies such as proton pump inhibitors supports the role of bile aspiration, not acid reflux underpinning this lung damage. A pervasive microbial signature, strongly dominated by pathogenic proteobacterial species, in the lungs of CF patients has been described with both the biodiversity and community structure correlating with patients disease status and lung function. The lung microbiome in bile aspirating patients was consistent with this pervasive microbial signature, whilst the community profiles of non-aspirating CF patients were consistent with that of healthy non-CF individuals (Reen et al. 2014, Blainey et al. 2012, Cox et al. 2010). This is the first evidence implicating aspirated bile in shaping the CF lung microbiome and encouraging disease progression. A possible insight into how this aspirated bile promotes the emergence of pathogenic proteobacteria in the lung comes from recent studies demonstrating the effect of bile on individual respiratory pathogens. The dominant CF pathogen *Pseudomonas aeruginosa*, upregulated phenotypes commonly associated with chronic infection such as biofilm formation and quorum sensing when exposed to bile while phenotypes associated with acute infection were repressed (Reen et al. 2012). This further suggests that bile is a major host determinant with a significant role in signaling bacteria to switch to a chronic lifestyle.

These new findings, in what is a relatively new and dynamic area of research, hold significant clinical potential for the improvement of both the treatments available and the quality of life of CF patients. It is ultimately hoped that a better understanding of how bile mediates the development of chronic infections can translate into better clinical management of CF.

ABBREVIATIONS

CF	Cystic Fibrosis
COPD	Chronic Obstructive Pulmonary Disease
WHO	World Health Organisation
BALF	Bronchoalveolar lavage fluid
FEV	Forced expiratory volume
GOR	Gastro-oesophageal reflux
GORD	Gatro-oesophageal reflux disease
PPI	Proton pump inhibitors
LOS	Lower oesophageal sphincter
T3SS	Type three secretion system
T6SS	Type six secretion system
PQS	Pseudomonas Quinolone signal

CHRONIC RESPIRATORY DISEASE

Chronic respiratory diseases, including Cystic Fibrosis (CF), Chronic Obstructive Pulmonary Disease (COPD), asthma, idiopathic pulmonary fibrosis and non CF-Bronchiectasis, are rapidly emerging as a global health problem. These diseases are amongst the leading causes of death worldwide and represent a significant social and economic burden in terms of public health costs. These costs are primarily due to the expenses associated with long term disease management and loss of productivity due to disability. In the European Union (EU) alone the annual cost of respiratory disease is greater than €380 billion with an estimated €48.4 billion due to COPD and €33.9 billion due to asthma. The economic costs associated with CF are estimated to be €600 million per annum by the European Respiratory Society (ERS) and with the advent of new and expensive therapeutics will be expected to increase substantially (European Respiratory Society, 2015).

Whilst the underlying pathophysiology of these respiratory diseases is unique, disease progression is often mediated by chronic infection or chronic inflammation which is accompanied by a gradual loss of lung function (Nichols et al. 2008, Sethi et al. 2009). In fact, for COPD, CF and non CF-bronchiectasis, the "vicious cycle" hypothesis has been proposed whereby infection or inhalation of toxic substances, such as tobacco smoke, impairs the innate immune system within the lung.

This induces an overt immune response resulting in chronic inflammation which perpetuates chronic airway infection (Sethi et al. 2009, Nichols et al. 2008, Altenburg et al. 2015).

Pathophysiology of CF

These chronic airway infections are a leading cause of morbidity and mortality, particularly within the CF population. As much of the primary research regarding bile aspiration has been carried out in a CF cohort, much of the emphasis will be placed on this condition. However, the reported findings may be applicable to the spectrum of respiratory disease described in this review but requires further investigation. CF is the most common autosomal recessive genetic disease within the Caucasian population, affecting more than 70,000 people worldwide. This genetic condition is caused by a mutation in the Cystic Fibrosis Conductance Regulator (CFTR) protein encoding an Adenosine Triphosphate (ATP) driven chloride pump (Gibson et al. 2003). The mutation produces a defective CFTR protein which impairs normal airway clearance and results in an accumulation of viscous mucus within the lungs. This mucus is a favourable environment for both commensal and pathogenic microorganisms which are capable of causing airway infections. This results in the generation of an overt immune response culminating in prolonged inflammation in the lungs (Lynch and Bruce 2013, Zemanick et al. 2011) (Table 1). Whether these airway infections are the initial driver of inflammation is still under investigation (Rao and Grigg 2006). Inflammation of the lungs has been detected in paediatric patients before the onset of infection highlighting the importance of other determinants in the pathophysiology of CF (Schultz and Stick 2015, Khan et al. 1995).

Pathophysiology of COPD and Other Respiratory Diseases

COPD is a life-threatening lung disease, characterized by severe limitations in lung airflow with a progressive decline in lung function. The primary cause of this disease is excessive direct or indirect tobacco smoke, and although preventable, COPD cannot be cured (Table 1). The World Health Organization estimates that 64 million people have COPD where 3 million people die from the disease every year (WHO, 2015).

Table 1. Outlined below are the primary clinical symptoms and pathophysiology underlying selected chronic respiratory conditions. These conditions are mediated by either chronic infection or chronic inflammation and in some, combinations of both which leads to a progressive loss of lung function

Respiratory Disease	Pathophysiology
Cystic Fibrosis	• Chronic infection and inflammation • Chronic *Pseudomonas aeruginosa* infection accompanied by loss in biodiversity of microbial communities • Gradual loss of pulmonary function
Chronic Obstructive Pulmonary Disease	• Chronic Inflammation and fibrosis of airways • Progressive loss of lung function • Variable disease severity- Global initiative for chronic obstructive pulmonary disease (GOLD) classification
Asthma	• Autoimmune disease • Chronic inflammation due to bronchial hyper responsiveness • Long term airway remodelling
Idiopathic Pulmonary Fibrosis	• Autoimmune or infection induced lung damage • Chronic inflammation • Impaired wound healing response and fibrosis of lower airways
Non-CF Bronchiectasis	• Chronic infection and inflammation • Dysfunctional immune system • Abnormal dilation of the walls of the bronchi

While COPD affects both the innate and adaptive immune processes, disease progression is characterized by increased pulmonary inflammation and accelerated by acute exacerbations usually precipitated by persistent or acute respiratory infections. Several pathogens are associated with exacerbations in COPD including *Haemophilus influenza*, *Streptococcus pneumonia*, *Moraxella catarrhalis* and most importantly *Pseudomonas aeruginosa*. *P. aeruginosa* is one of the most commonly occurring pathogens in COPD, causing both acute and chronic infections, it is often found in patients with more severe symptoms and is associated with increased mortality (Almagro et al. 2012, Hassett et al. 2014).

This persistent airway inflammation and destruction is also evident in other respiratory diseases such as asthma, idiopathic pulmonary fibrosis and non CF-bronchiectasis (Table 1). Asthma is an inflammatory disease characterized by air flow obstruction and bronchial hyper-responsiveness which is estimated to affect >230 million people worldwide (ERS, 2015). In asthma inflammation and bronchial obstruction results from a hyper sensitivity to numerous stimuli. This results in mononuclear cell and eosinophil infiltration and mucus hyper secretion. It is becoming clear that microbial infections can also play a part in the pathophysiology of asthma. Several pathogens including *Chlamydia pneumoniae*, *Mycoplasma pneumoniae* and *Staphylococcus aureus* have been associated with increased exacerbations in asthma patients whilst *H. influenzae*, *M. catarrhalis* and *Streptococcus pneumoniae* have been linked to increased morbidity (Guilbert and Denlinger 2010, Redinbo 2014, Korppi 2010). *H. influenzae* in particular has been found to be associated with neutrophilic asthma, a form of asthma where inflammation is mainly mediated by neutrophils (Korppi 2010).

REFRACTORY NATURE OF CHRONIC RESPIRATORY DISEASE

A variety of treatments exists for the daily management of these respiratory conditions in an attempt to improve the quality of life of affected individuals. These treatments primarily focus on a combination of chest physiotherapy to clear excess mucus from the lungs, the use of bronchodilators and corticosteroids to relieve symptoms of breathlessness and intensive antibiotic therapy to control frequent airway infections (Barnes 2011, Main et al. 2015, Weiner et al. 2008). However, whilst patient life expectancy and quality of life has undoubtedly improved, these conventional therapies are largely ineffective in modulating disease progression where in cases of severe lung damage a patient may be required to undergo lung transplantation. This is further confounded by the fact that antibiotics become largely redundant once respiratory pathogens adopt a chronic biofilm lifestyle where bacteria become tolerant to many antibiotics (Hoiby et al. 2010). Furthermore, the rapid spread of antibiotic resistance through bacterial populations resulting in multi drug resistant pathogens means many antibiotics are becoming ineffective in the control of infectious disease particularly pulmonary disease (McGowan 2006). Similarly, the rate of novel antibiotic discovery has significantly declined announcing the arrival of a post antibiotic era. Financial constraints in industry mean novel antimicrobial discovery is no longer a priority with calls for redesign of the antibiotics pipeline (Lewis 2013, Aminov, World Health Organisation 2014, Cooper and Shlaes 2011). These developments signify the urgent need for alternatives to antibiotics.

Whilst the development of these chronic respiratory diseases is multifactorial the interaction between the host and colonising microbes is fundamental to the pathophysiology of disease progression. Therefore, it follows that a potential alternative strategy could emerge from the study of the microbiology of chronic respiratory disease, particularly how respiratory pathogens residing in the lung are triggered to adopt a chronic biofilm lifestyle.

MONITORING THE LUNG MICROBIOME IN RESPIRATORY DISEASE PATIENTS

Several studies have confirmed the microbiological basis of chronic pulmonary disease and have revealed that both the lungs of healthy and diseased individuals harbour diverse communities of bacteria and are not sterile environments as was previously believed (Beck et al. 2012, Charlson et al. 2012a, Charlson et al. 2012b, Erb-Downward 2012, Sibley et al. 2006, Hilty et al. 2010). A comprehensive knowledge of the differences between microbial communities (known as the microbiome) residing in the lungs of healthy and diseased patients could further enhance our understanding of their role in the progression of respiratory disease. Additionally, insights into the influence of host physiological factors that shape these dynamic populations could further aid the design of novel therapeutic plans.

Sampling Techniques for the Identification and Characterization of the Lung Microbiome

To examine these microbial communities the lung environment must first be sampled with specific consideration to the location of sampling and the level of invasiveness (Proctor 2011). There are four types of sample that can be used; 1) bronchoalveolar lavage fluid (BALF), 2) induced or expectorated sputum sampling, 3) deep throat swab and 4) sampling of the explanted lung

(Erb-Downward 2012) summarised in table 2 below. BALF, the gold standard for sampling the lung microbiome environment, is obtained during a lung bronchoscopy where various areas of the lung can be sampled (Harris et al. 2007, Charlson et al. 2011, Twigg et al. 2013). In adults, this procedure is minimally invasive only requiring the administration of local anaesthetic and sedative whilst in paediatric patients this procedure is considerably more invasive as general anaesthetic is required with an increased risk of trauma to the airway epithelium (Roberts and Thornington 2005). As many microbiome studies encompass paediatric patients, the level of invasiveness should be a primary consideration when choosing a sample type. Furthermore, this option can often become prohibitively expensive for use on a wide scale basis in large clinical cohorts (Choure et al. 2005).

The preferred alternative to BALF is the use of expectorated or induced sputum samples. Sputum comprises the thick mucus that is coughed up by patients from the lower airways; expectorated sputum is generated solely by coughing whilst induced sputum requires the inhalation of a hypertonic saline solution. The use of sputum, both expectorated and induced, has many advantages; it is safe, non-invasive, can be routinely carried out and is inexpensive (Mussaffi et al. 2008). Therefore it is the most widely practiced technique of sampling the lung microbiota.

Table 2. The advantages and disadvantages associated with sample types employed in the study of the lung environment. There is a trade-off between samples that are most representative

Sample type	Advantages	Disadvantages
Bronchoalveolar lavage fluid	Gold standard for sampling	Expensive as it can require the use of anaesthetic, invasive in paediatrics
Sputum—Induced —Expectorated	Minimally invasive so can be carried out routinely	Risk of contamination by the upper respiratory tract
Deep throat swab	Can be carried out routinely and inexpensively	Not always representative of the lower airway microbiome
Explanted lung	Can sample several areas	Only available following lung transplantation in patients with severe disease

The primary disadvantage associated with the use of sputum is the potential risk of cross-contamination by microbial communities present in the upper respiratory tract (Goddard et al. 2012). However, several recent studies have identified distinct microbial communities in the oropharyngeal tract when compared to that of the lower respiratory microbiome with minimal cross contamination (Rogers et al. 2006, Blainey et al. 2012, Boutin et al. 2015). In patients exhibiting stable respiratory disease, the microbiome of the throat and lung harbour similar microbial communities whilst the microbiomes of those exhibiting severe disease are increasingly dissimilar. Deep throat swabs could therefore be employed as a means of sampling the lung environment in clinically stable patients (Boutin et al. 2015). Lastly, in patients with end stage lung disease who may have to undergo lung transplantation, microbial sampling of the explanted lungs can be carried out. Analysis of these microbial communities further confirmed that BAL and sputum are an effective means of sampling the lung environment (Erb-Downward et al. 2011).

What has become increasingly apparent in microbiome analysis is that the use of culture dependent techniques alone is insufficient in providing a fully representative overview of the complexity of microbial communities present. The primary limitation of culturing is that only a percentage (1%) of the bacteria can be cultivated. This phenomenon was coined the "plate count anomaly" by Staley and Konopka in 1985 to describe the apparent inability to culture many microbes visible under the microscope (Staley and Konopka 1985). To culture this 1% is both challenging and time consuming (Bittar and Rolain 2010). However, a study by Sibley et al. demonstrated that the majority of bacteria present in the CF airway are readily cultured through an enrichment of conventional microbiology techniques. With a combination of culture dependent and culture independent techniques increasing the sensitivity of detection of bacteria within the CF lung (Sibley et al. 2011). The advances in culture independent techniques in recent years has provided a better understanding of the complexity of the human microbiota (Aho et al. 2015, Berger et al. 2015, Ursell et al. 2012). Next Generation Sequencing (NGS) including 454 sequencing, Illumina HiSeq and MiSeq and PacBio has become more affordable allowing increased species level identification offering a more representative view of the lung microbiome (Armougom et al. 2009, Kuczynski et al. 2011). The emergence of third generation sequencing technologies such as Oxford nanopore technologies and ion torrent require just a single molecule of DNA to sequence which could potentially translate into faster and cheaper sequencing of lung microbiomes (Schadt et al. 2010).

The availability of such a wide array of technology means studies conducted on the lung environment generates a vast amount of information. Comparisons between studies should be interpreted cautiously as standardised practices have yet to be established. Variablity exists in the choice of sample type, method of DNA extraction and sequencing technology; all of which can introduce biases into microbiome studies. Hence what is critical for this rapidly emerging field is the design of standardised practices, an issue that must be addressed for future research. Nevertheless, microbiome studies have been conducted for many respiratory conditions with a pervasive microbiome reported for CF that has been correlated with patient disease status (Blainey et al. 2012). Signature microbiome profiles are currently being investigated for COPD, asthma and bronchiectasis (Aguirre et al. 2015, Huang and Boushey 2015).

A Pervasive Microbiome Exists in CF Patients

The lungs of CF patients harbour diverse microbial communities with independent studies detecting up to 100 genera of bacteria (Cox et al. 2010, Madan et al. 2012, Guss et al. 2011). This is significantly more diverse than previously estimated and is an unsurprising fact, as the CF lung is a warm, humid environment, organically rich and when defective in mucociliary clearance, microbial communities can proliferate exponentially without removal. The CF lung is therefore a favourable niche for microbial communities to exploit (Worlitzsch et al. 2002, Matsui et al. 2006, Guss et al. 2011). CF has been identified as a polymicrobial disease where pulmonary exacerbations, described as a temporary decline in lung function, are driven by multiple microbial species. This means that treatment strategies based solely on the identification of pathogenic bacteria through routine culturing are now becoming ineffective (Sibley et al. 2006, Sibley et al. 2008, Sibley et al. 2011, Rogers et al. 2004). Whilst, the microbiome is relatively constant in clinically stable patients, patients experiencing an exacerbation display dynamic changes in community structure with no significant change in bacterial load. This highlights the importance of community diversity in the maintenance of lung health (Stokell et al. 2015, Carmody et al. 2013, Carmody et al. 2015). The "Keystone pathogen hypothesis" could explain this observation. This attempts to describe the role of polymicrobial interactions within the lung whereby low abundance members of the community such as the recently identified *Gemella* genera, play a major role in the remodelling of the microbiota to that of a dysbiotic pathogenic community (Hajishengallis et al. 2011, Carmody et al. 2013, Hajishengallis et al. 2012). Even with the emergence of new treatments such as Ivacaftor (Kapoor et al. 2014, Wainwright et al. 2015, Flume et al. 2012) which have revolutionised CF treatments, understanding the CF microbiome in terms of both low and high abundance genera remains a key research question. Particularly, as those receiving treatment will have a degree of pre-existing airway destruction and an increased risk of infection (Flume and Van Devanter 2012, Surette 2014).

Both genetic and environmental factors have been shown to influence the composition of the CF lung via sibling and twin studies (Collaco et al. 2010, Hampton et al. 2014, Stressmann et al. 2011). At the phylum level, the majority of the genera belong to Proteobacteria, Bacteroidetes, Fusobacteria and Firmicutes (Guss et al. 2011, Cox et al. 2010). A signature CF microbiome has been described which is heavily dominated by the routinely culturable CF pathogens; *Pseudomonas aeruginosa, Staphylococcus aureus, Haemophilus influenza and Burkholderia cepacia* complex (Blainey et al. 2012, Gibson et al. 2003, Surette 2014, Lynch and Bruce 2013). However these pathogenic bacteria represent a tiny portion of the total microbiome. Improvements in clinical management protocols have been effective in the control of common respiratory pathogens. However, new multidrug resistant pathogens such as *Achrobacter* species, *Stenotrophomas maltophilia* and *Streptococcus milleri* are now emerging for which new molecular therapies are required (Mahenthiralingam 2014). However the role of the *Streptococcus milleri* group in pulmonary exacerbations is still controversial as there are varying reports regarding their abundance and correlation with disease status (Parkins et al. 2008, Carmody et al. 2013, Filkins et al. 2012) Whilst a signature CF microbiome exists there is high inter-individual variation with individuals harbouring personal microbiomes. Personalised medical strategies could potentially exploit the existence of unique microbiomes through probiotic manipulation (Nagalingam et al. 2013, Gollwitzer and Marsland 2014). Interestingly, the lung microbiome contains a relatively high proportion of anaerobic bacteria particularly *Streptococcus, Rothia, Veillonella, Prevotella* and *Porphyromonas* are opportunistic pathogens and may be of clinical value (Guss et al. 2011, Tunney et al. 2008). The presence of anaerobes may be explained by the thick mucus environment within the lung which is anoxic in nature due to slow diffusion of oxygen and rapid utilisation of available sources by aerobic bacteria. This mechanism generates anaerobic and microaerophilic pockets in the lungs which are occupied by both strict and facultative anaerobes (Worlitzsch et al. 2002, Matsui et al. 2006, Alvarez-

Ortega and Harwood 2007). This heterogeneity within the lung environment is reflected in the variation of community structure and composition depending on the location of sampling. This spatial heterogeneity has been proposed to explain the variability in sputum samples obtained from the same individual, further highlighting the necessity for standardised protocols (Willner et al. 2012). The discovery that strict anaerobes are commonly present in the CF lungs also points to the limitations of conventional microbiology as these categories of bacteria are difficult to culture in a clinical setting (Tunney et al. 2008).

Findings from numerous cross sectional studies have revealed progressive increases in the diversity of bacterial communities as a patient ages, however, as patients transition to adulthood, there is a gradual decrease in diversity where communities become dominated by a single pathogenic species. Recent studies have shown this process is largely completed by the age of 25 (Cox et al. 2010, Coburn et al. 2015). Pathogenic domination of the CF lung is largely due to *Pseudomonas aeruginosa,* which chronically infects up to 80% of CF patients (Davies 2002, Pressler et al. 2011). Environmental conditions within the lung such as reduced oxygen tension promotes the outgrowth of *Pseudomonas aeruginosa.* Chronic infection by *P. aeruginosa* is correlated with a lower forced expiratory volume (FEV), a clinical measurement of lung function (Davies 2002, Staudinger et al. 2014). There is also evidence of early homeostatic disruption to the CF lung when compared to healthy controls, indicating a fundamental disturbance at an early age (Renwick et al. 2014). This trend towards reduced microbial diversity is characterised by a reduction in evenness and richness of microbial populations and is negatively correlated with clinical status and pulmonary function. This observation is becoming a predominant feature of many chronic inflammatory conditions (Comito et al. 2014, Levy 2012). Furthermore, microbial communities in older patients are composed of more phylogenetically related populations which are potentially resistant to antimicrobial treatment strategies (Cox et al. 2010, Flanagan et al. 2007). Whilst data generated from these studies are informative they are significantly limited by their cross sectional study design and small sample size (McDonald et al. 2015, Carmody et al. 2015). A concerted shift to longitudinal analyses and clinical follow-up would be more useful in the long term as these studies would provide insights into microbiome evolution with respect to patient aging.

Chronic infection of the CF lung by pathogenic bacteria is a primary indicator of poor clinical prognosis. This is predominantly due to the ability of these bacteria to adopt a biofilm mode of growth which is refractive to antibiotic therapy (Hoiby et al. 2010). It is clear from the above that the microbiome is profoundly shaped by clinical intervention. Though the importance of host factors in disease progression has yet to be fully established. Knowledge of the role of host factors is vital to understanding the means through which remodelling of the CF microbiome occurs. As well as the means by which pathogenic bacteria emerge to chronically dominate the local community.

The COPD Microbiome

Similar to the pathology observed in CF, overproduction of mucus in COPD creates a niche environment for microorganisms increasing the risk of recurrent airway/lung infections. These airway infections have been associated with the accelerated rate of lung function decline in COPD (Vestbo et al. 1996, Kanner et al. 2001). The COPD lung harbours diverse communities of bacteria which includes the routinely cultured *Streptococcus, Moraxella* and *Haemophilus* genera these are the primary pathogens associated with COPD pulmonary infections (Han et al. 2012, Huang et al. 2010). However, other genera such as *Veillonella, Actinomyces, Neisseria, Prevotella, Gemella* and *Rothia* may potentially be implicated in the pathophysiology of this disease (Millares et al. 2014). Importantly, no significant difference has been observed in the diversity or relative abundance of bacteria present between COPD patients and that of non-COPD control subjects (Erb-Downward et al. 2011, Huang et al. 2010) However, early in COPD disease progression, a distinct microbial composition emerges (Sze et al. 2012, Pragman et al. 2012). Whilst some studies report a marked reduction in microbial diversity in patients exhibiting moderate to severe disease, others report a correlation between increase diversity and disease status. It has therefore been suggested that there are two possible distinct microbiomes associated with COPD. A Proteobacterial dominated microbiome associated with low bacterial diversity and a Firmicutes dominated microbiome associated with higher bacterial diversity (Erb-Downward et al. 2011, Sze et al. 2012, Huang et al. 2010, Hilty et al. 2010). However, the inconsistencies in the literature mean no definitive evidence exists establishing the link between diversity levels and disease severity. Furthermore unlike in CF where loss of diversity accompanies outgrowth of a pathogenic species, COPD does not appear to yield a dominant genera. Further microbiome analysis of the COPD lung is required in order to fully characterise the microbiological basis underpinning the pathology of this disease. Future studies may shed some light on the apparent variability in the published results. A possible reason for the inconsistencies in the data between research groups could be due to the lack of uniform and standardised protocols for lung microbiome analysis as described above. Most significantly the use of different control groups when carrying out comparisons, further highlighting the central importance of experimental design when undertaking microbiome analysis.

HOST FACTORS MODULATING RESPIRATORY DISEASE PROGRESSION

It is clear therefore, that there is a microbiological basis underlying several chronic respiratory conditions with a pervasive microbiome identified for CF and emerging microbiomes for COPD and asthma. The frequent pulmonary exacerbations resulting from disruptions to the structures of these communities are associated with increased morbidity and mortality in respiratory cohorts (Carmody et al. 2013, Carmody et al. 2015). This vicious cycle of chronic infection and inflammation cannot be controlled resulting in progressive respiratory decline. As a result there have been investigations attempting to identify environmental or host factors correlating with disease progression and clinical outcome (Nichols et al. 2008, Papi et al. 2006). These investigations led to the discovery of a correlation between gastro-oesophageal reflux disease (GORD) and chronic respiratory disease. GORD (GERD in the US) was found to be a major co-morbidity of CF and COPD (Reen et al. 2012, Reen et al. 2014, Samareh Fekri et al. 2013, Sweet et al. 2009). In patients diagnosed with GORD, a variety of pulmonary manifestations could be observed such as chronic cough, bronchitis, bronchial asthma, bronchitis, pneumonia and interstitial fibrosis (Gaude 2009). This led to the suggestions that GORD is an underlying host factor of chronic respiratory disease though the exact mechanism through which it elicits this effect remains unknown.

Co-Morbidity of GORD with Lung Disease

The co-morbidity of GORD with chronic respiratory disease is now widely accepted however the mechanisms through which the lung damage is incurred has yet to be elucidated. It was first proposed in 1975 that GORD contributes to progressive lung decline with GORD positive patients exhibiting more severe respiratory disease (Feigelson, J. 1975). The incidence of GORD is estimated to be as high as 80% in CF patients and up to 40% of COPD patients (Pauwels et al. 2012). However, this figure may be an underestimation of the prevalence within these populations due to limitations in diagnosis of GORD which will be further discussed below. GORD is a condition resulting in the returning of the contents of the stomach in to the oesophagus. It is ultimately a clinical manifestation resulting from a disruption to a normal physiological process where barriers that control reflux are impaired and no longer function effectively (Button et al. 2005, Patrick 2011). Comprising three broad categories, GORD is a spectrum disease where patients exhibit mild to severe disease symptoms; i) non-erosive reflux disease, where there is no evidence of mucosal damage, ii) erosive esophagitis and iii) Barrett's oesophagus, where there is evidence of damage to the mucosa (Sontag et al. 2006, Agrawal and Castell 2006). Many physiological risk factors contribute to GORD development, such as a defective lower oesophageal sphincter (LOS), increased lower abdominal pressure and delayed gastric emptying. These symptoms are commonly present in patients with underlying respiratory conditions such as CF and COPD. GORD is further enhanced by daily chest physiotherapy treatment regimens. Typically diagnosis depends on presentation with clinical symptoms such as heartburn, acid regurgitation and stomach pain however, up to 50% of patients do not present with these characteristic symptoms making clinical diagnosis a challenge (Scott and Gelhot 1999, Button et al. 2005, Blondeau et al. 2010, Vakil et al. 2006) Furthermore, GOR diagnosis is exacerbated by asymptomatic or silent GOR, therefore diagnosis based solely on symptomatic presentation is limited with recommendations that patients be monitored and tested for reflux.

Clinical Diagnosis of GOR

Clinically, several methods are used to test for GORD including endoscopy, manometry, proton pump inhibitor testing (PPI), and multichannel intraluminal impedance pH monitoring. Endoscopic diagnosis investigating mucosal damage is routinely used but has low sensitivity of detection (Lichtenstein et al. 2007). Alternatively, manometry is effective in the analysis of oesophageal and LOS functioning but is conventionally performed in the evaluation of a patient's suitability for anti-reflux surgery (Akyuz et al. 2009).

PPI testing is an ineffective strategy for the diagnosis of GORD due to subjectivity. This involves the prescription of PPI drugs to affected patients where diagnosis is based solely on symptomatic resolution (DeVault and Castell 2005). The gold standard for accurate diagnosis of GORD is intraluminal oesophageal impedance pH monitoring which detects both acid and non-acid reflux. The procedure involves placing a pH catheter into the oesophagus and monitoring pH over 24 hours (Mousa et al. 2011). Alternatively, the use of exhaled breath condensate for the detection of biomarkers such as pepsin is currently under investigation as a diagnostic tool for GORD (Lee et al. 2015).

BILE ASPIRATION: A UNIFYING PRINCIPAL UNDERLYING THE PATHOPHYSIOLOGY OF RESPIRATORY DISEASE

As a result of the correlation between GORD and lung function decline, it has been hypothesised that aspiration of bile into the respiratory tract is responsible for GORD induced lung damage. Bile is a component of the gastric contents that is refluxed during episodes of GOR. Indeed, physiologically relevant concentrations of bile have been shown to induce lung damage and inflammation in lung epithelial cells in culture (Legendre et al. 2014). The rate of bile aspiration is estimated to be as high as 80% in the CF population whilst the incidence of aspiration in other respiratory conditions should be further investigated. Aspiration of bile into the lungs has been shown via the detection of bile acids in BALF and sputum of respiratory patients (Reen et al. 2012, Aseeri et al. 2012, Neujahr et al. 2014, Blondeau et al. 2008a). Further evidence for the role of bile aspiration in lung disease has been observed in patients undergoing lung transplantation (Blondeau et al. 2008b). Bile acids have been detected in BALF samples from these patients following lung transplantation. Aspiration of bile has been indicated as a major risk factor for the development of bronchiolitis obliterans syndrome resulting in lung transplant rejection and increased colonisation with *P. aeruginosa* in these patients (Mertens et al. 2011, D'Ovidio et al. 2005). Administration of the macrolide antibiotic azithromycin to lung transplant recipients has reduced the level of aspiration improving clinical outcome. Mechanistically, it is proposed these antibiotics function through accelerated gastric emptying, however, their role in the control of GORD and bile aspiration in respiratory disease requires further investigation (Mertens et al. 2009).

Quantification and Profiling of Bile Acids in the Lungs

In order to assess patients effectively for bile aspiration, high resolution technologies for the detection of bile must be designed. Detection techniques have evolved from methods based on bile acid identification in other matrices such as blood. Currently, there is a lack of protocols in the literature describing the direct identification of bile acids from lung fluids, therefore advancements in this area are required to fully rationalize the emerging role of bile acid aspiration in chronic lung disease.

The utilization of an enzymatic reaction using 3-α hydroxysteroid dehydrogenase (3-α HSD) linked to colorimetric analysis to measure total bile acid levels from bronchoalveolar lavage (BAL) samples has been described (Niu 2014). 3-α HSD catalyzes the oxidation of the hydroxyl group at position 3 of the steroid ring. In the presence of the coenzyme nicotinamide adenine dinucleotide (NAD) 3-α HSD converts bile acids into 3-keto steroids and NADH which reacts with nitrotetrazolium blue in the presence of the diaphorase enzyme to form the dye, formazan, measured colorimetrically at O.D. 495_{nm}. Thus, total bile acids concentration can be calculated. Using this enzymatic approach, aspirated bile acids have been successfully identified in the lungs following transplantation and increased levels have been linked to the development of bronchiolitis obliterans syndrome (D'Ovidio et al. 2005).

While enzymatic assays are useful in giving total bile acids, major fluctuations in bile acid profiles may escape detection using this technique. High resolution liquid chromatography–mass spectrometry (LC-MS) is currently one of the most accurate technology for the quantification of bile acids. Most methods rely on reverse phase chromatography with a variety of flow rates and column dimensions (Roda et al. 1995, Goto et al. 2007). LC-MS (and MS/MS) detects bile acids from a number of different matrices including, blood serum (Burkard et al. 2005), human bile (Perwaiz et al. 2001), stool (Kakiyama et al. 2014) and the brain (Mano et al. 2004). To confront bile aspiration and its influence on chronic respiratory infection, a highly sensitive and specific LC-MS method was developed (Reen et al. 2014). This method has been successfully applied to the analysis of sputum samples from a cohort of pediatric CF patients for the detection and accurate profiling of bile acids. Aspirated bile acid has also been measured in airway secretions collected from intubated and mechanically ventilated patients. The increased bile acid levels were shown to be associated with detrimental ventilator-associated pneumonia (Wu et al. 2009). Direct electrospray ionization mass spectrometry can also be utilized successfully to identify bile acids in the lower airways of adult CF patients with robust detection limits (0.01 μmol/L) (Aseeri et al. 2012). However, it has been suggested this method is not the most suitable for many biological matrices due to their complexity (Griffiths and Sjövall 2009). Studies investigating the potential use of exhaled breath condensate for the diagnosis of bile aspiration are currently underway. However, there are limitations with regard to the sensitivity of detection and diagnostic value as it is just an indicator of GORD (Reder et al. 2014).

Aspirated Bile Shapes the CF Microbiome

The existence of a pervasive CF microbiome, along with emerging evidence for a COPD microbiome has prompted several microbiome investigations delineating the role of bile in the aspirated lung of CF patients. A study carried out in our laboratory has demonstrated physiologically relevant concentrations of bile were present in the sputum of paediatric CF patients (Reen et al. 2014). Stratification of patients based on their aspiration status revealed a significant reduction in biodiversity and richness levels triggering the emergence of dominant Proteobacterial pathogens as seen in Figure 1 below. Interestingly, patients classified as non-aspirating had a much greater microbial biodiversity with microbiomes more closely resembling that of a healthy non CF lung. Aspirating patients displayed the pervasive CF microbiome containing dominant Proteobacterial genera such as *Pseudomonas, Stenotrophomonas* and *Ralstonia* which when present could account for up to 98% of the microbial sample (Reen et al. 2014). These findings mirrored previous studies examining CF vs non CF patients and indicated that stratification of respiratory cohorts based on aspiration status must be a consideration in future microbiome studies, particularly in the emerging COPD and asthma microbiomes (Blainey et al. 2012). Furthermore, bile could potentially shape the two distinct microbiomes observed in COPD, one dominated by the Proteobacterial phylum as in aspirating CF patients and one dominated by the Firmicutes phylum as in non-aspirating CF patients (Huang et al. 2010). This initial pilot study by Reen et al. firmly established bile as a major host factor shaping the respiratory microbiome which in turn could have a significant impact on the progression of respiratory disease. The strong correlation between bile acid aspiration with biodiversity and the prevalence of CF associated pathogens warrants further investigation particularly longitudinal analysis.

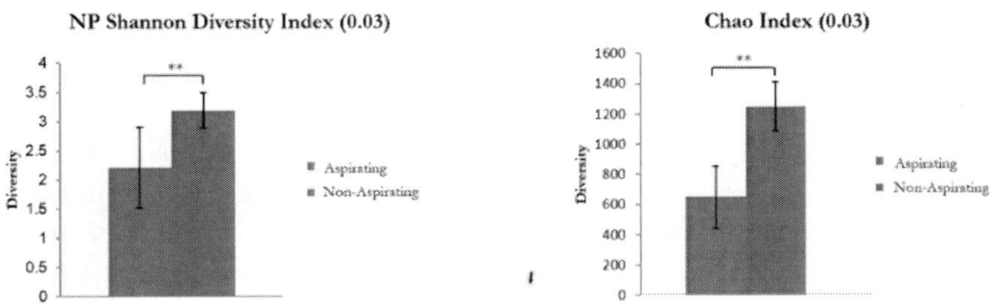

Family level relative abundance

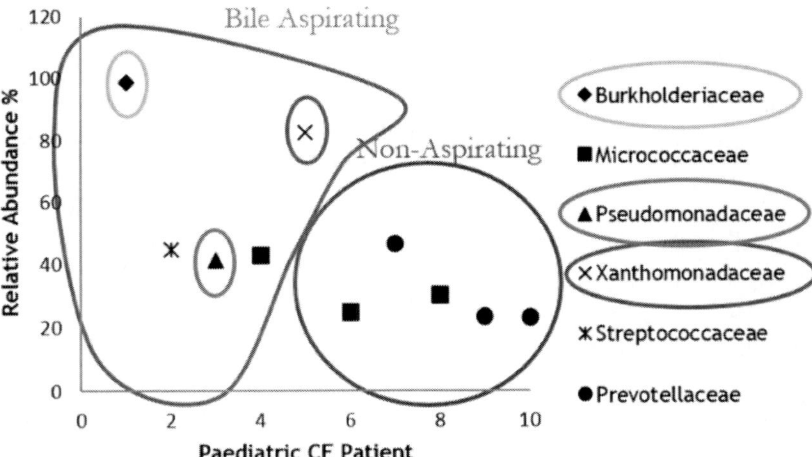

Adapted from Reen et al. 2014.

Figure 1. Aspirating patients display a reduction in both biodiversity and richness (Shannon and Chao index) with an emergence of Proteobacterial pathogens such as members of the family Burkholderiaceae and Pseudomonadaceae.

Bile Triggers Respiratory Pathogens to Adopt a Chronic Lifestyle

While bile acid signaling has long been associated with a broad spectrum of diseases such as diabetes, gastrointestinal disease and obesity (Jones et al. 2014). The possibility that bile is potentially a signaling molecule in respiratory disease had not previously been considered. The strong correlation between the presence of aspirated bile and the emergence of dominant Proteobacterial pathogens within the CF lung microbiome suggests that bile might impact directly on the behavior of the pathogen itself.

Studies on the influence of bile on the human microbiota have been restricted to enteric pathogens associated with gastroenteritis and gut infections as well as probiotics, and have focused largely on their capacity for bile tolerance (Begley et al. 2005, Merritt and Donaldson 2009, Patel et al. 2010, Koskenniemi et al. 2011). However, enteric bacteria would appear to employ species-specific mechanisms in response to exogenous bile. For instance, the Type 3 Secretion System (T3SS) was reduced in *Salmonella enterica* in response to bile (Prouty and Gunn 2000), while it was increased in *Shigella flexneri*, *Vibrio parahaemolyticus* (Olive et al. 2007, Gotoh et al. 2010, Barta et al. 2012) and in the protozoan pathogen Cryptosporidium spp (Feng et al. 2006). Furthermore, while motility was decreased in *S. enterica* it was increased in *V. cholera* (Gupta and Chowdhury 1997). Therefore, the impact of aspirated bile on the respiratory microbiota in the lung may be similarly diverse. Studies on the mechanisms underpinning the response of gastrointestinal bacteria to bile have recently led to the identification of a bile 'sensor' in *Listeria monocytogenes* (Quillin et al. 2011), while a role for two component systems has also been reported in *S. enterica* (Prouty et al. 2004). However, until recently, no information was available on the influence of bile on respiratory pathogens, which are likely to encounter reduced, non-toxic levels of bile depending on the bacteria through aspiration. This would be analogous to the recent finding that sub-inhibitory concentrations of antibiotics elicit specific adaptive responses in pathogens, distinct from the response to higher toxic levels (Cummins et al. 2009).

Consistent with the association between aspirated bile and Proteobacterial pathogens, bile, and specifically bile acids were shown to elicit a chronic persistent biofilm lifestyle in a broad spectrum of respiratory disease pathogens. Studies on *P. aeruginosa* in particular revealed that, once exposed to physiologically relevant concentrations of bile, the pathogen adopted a chronic lifestyle, suppressing virulence systems associated with the acute phase of infection, and adopting a signal rich biofilm mode of growth (Reen et al. 2012). This switch from acute to chronic is characteristic of *P. aeruginosa* behavior in respiratory diseases such as CF, where the chronic behavior of this primary pathogen underlies the morbidity and mortality that underpin the pathophysiology of this disease. Indeed, chronic infection by *P. aeruginosa* has been shown to be associated with a lower FEV in childhood, a faster decline in FEV despite optimal respiratory management, higher mortality rate and shorter median survival (Lee et al. 2003).

Once *P. aeruginosa* changes its lifestyle from an acute virulent phenotype to a chronic biofilm mode of growth clinical management through antibiotic administration becomes largely ineffective. Therefore, there is a critical need to understand the molecular mechanisms through which this and other respiratory pathogens adopt the chronic biofilm lifestyle.

However, whilst much is known about the molecular basis of this lifestyle switch as outlined in Figure 2, little is known about the environmental signals that trigger this switch. Identifying those signals could offer new alternative strategies for the management of respiratory infections whereby pathogens would be locked in the acute phase of infection and therefore susceptible to conventional antibiotics.

Although currently there is no universally accepted clinical definition of chronic *P. aeruginosa* infection (Pressler et al. 2011), the phenotypic changes that occur during the transition have been well characterized in this organism. The acute to chronic switch involves the suppression of key acute virulence determinants such as the Type three Secretion system (T3SS), phenazine production, and swarming motility, while the chronic persistent lifestyle is adopted through increased biofilm formation and the production of chronic virulence systems such as the Type six secretion system (T6SS). Coordinating this switch are several layers of regulation, including the quorum sensing (QS) signaling pathway, of which there are three in *P. aeruginosa*. *P. aeruginosa* encodes two classical acyl-homoserine lactone (AHL) QS systems (LasIR and RhlIR), as well as an alkyl quinolone (AQ) system controlled by the Pseudomonas Quinolone Signal (PQS) and its precursor HHQ.

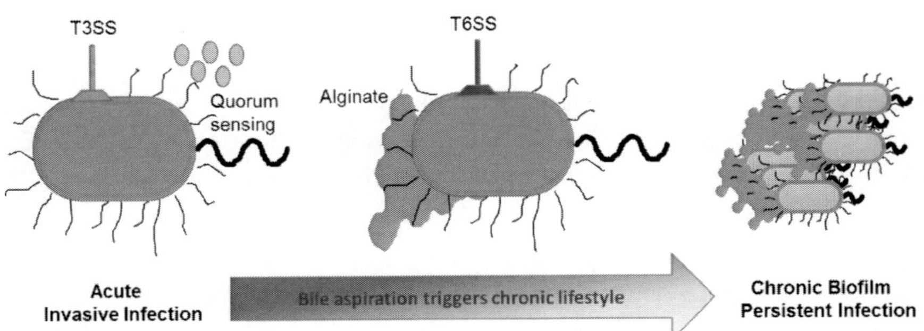

Figure 2. The molecular mechanism underlying *Pseudomonas aeruginosa* lifestyle switch from an acute, virulent lifestyle which encompasses the activity of the Type three Secretion system and quorum sensing to a chronic, persistent infection involving biofilm production and Type six secretion. Bile may be a major host factor triggering this lifestyle switch.

All 3 of these systems are involved in cell to cell communication, and the alkyl quinolone system in particular, has previously been shown to have a role in biofilm formation and persistence (Yang et al. 2009).

Addition of exogenous bile significantly increased biofilm formation and repressed the swarming motility of *P. aeruginosa*. In addition, production of all three *P. aeruginosa* quorum sensing (QS) signals, which have been detected in biofilms and CF sputum (Singh et al. 2000, Guina et al. 2003, Bleves et al. 2005), was increased in the presence of bile (Reen et al. 2012). Furthermore, expression of the chronic associated T6SS (Potvin et al. 2003, Mougous et al. 2006) was induced 3-fold in response to bile, while the acute-associated T3SS (Frank 1997, Vallis et al. 1999, O'Callaghan et al. 2011, O'Callaghan et al. 2012) was repressed (Reen et al. 2012). Notably, biofilm formation and PQS signaling were increased and swarming motility was repressed in the presence of bile salts, perhaps an indication that this may be the active bile component underlying the chronic pathogen response (Reen et al. 2012, Reen…O'Gara unpublished data).

The impact of bile was not restricted to *P.* aeruginosa, and consistent with the inter-patient diversity observed in the microbiome study. Bile also influenced other respiratory pathogens such as *Burkholderia cepacia* complex, *Acinetobacter baumanii*, and the emerging pathogen *Pandoraea sputonum* towards a biofilm mode of growth (Reen et al. 2012). In contrast, exposure to bile appeared to strongly repress biofilm formation in some isolates of *Staphylococcus aureus* and *Stenotrophomonas maltophilia* typed strains (Reen et al. 2012). However, the phenotypic response of clinical isolates from both species have recently been tested and, in contrast to the typed strains, lung clinical isolates exhibited a different response, with *S. aureus* isolates also adopting the biofilm lifestyle in response to bile (Ulluwishewa et al. 2015). This suggests some form of bacterial adaptation to what is emerging as a major host signal underlying the pathophysiology of respiratory disease. These strain and species-specific effects could further explain the mechanism through which bile shapes the respiratory microbiome triggering the emergence of dominant Proteobacterial pathogens (Reen et al. 2012). It certainly supports the hypothesis that bile directly influences the lung microbiome through modulation of pathogen behavior. Indeed, the modulation of both PQS signaling and T6SS is highly significant in light of their role in interspecies and inter-kingdom communication (Reen et al. 2011, Reen et al. 2013, Reen et al. 2015, Basler et al. 2013). The changes in population dynamics observed in bile aspirating patients may likely arise from the dual action of bile itself and that of the bile induced interspecies signal molecules, although these interactions are sure to be complex and difficult to define. Figure 3 summarizes the overall impact that bile elicits in the lung.

NEW HORIZONS FOR THE CLINICAL MANAGEMENT OF RESPIRATORY DISEASE

The current treatment plans of choice for GORD focus on acid suppression therapy through the use of proton pump inhibitor (PPI) and Histamine 2 receptor antagonists also known as H2 blockers. Both function by interfering with the gastric acid secretion pathway. H2 blockers are most effective at decreasing secretion after meals and are useful in the treatment of mild forms of the disease. PPI's are much more potent and function through irreversible binding of the H^+K^+ATPase. Though daily therapy is the preferred treatment option which controls the majority of patients symptoms, up to 30% of patients do not respond to therapy and continue to experience symptoms (Thomson 2008, Dean et al. 2004, Rackoff et al. 2005). As the rate of refractory GORD is so high and those receiving PPI treatment can still exhibit respiratory decline, alternative therapeutic management strategies must be sought for the control of GORD.

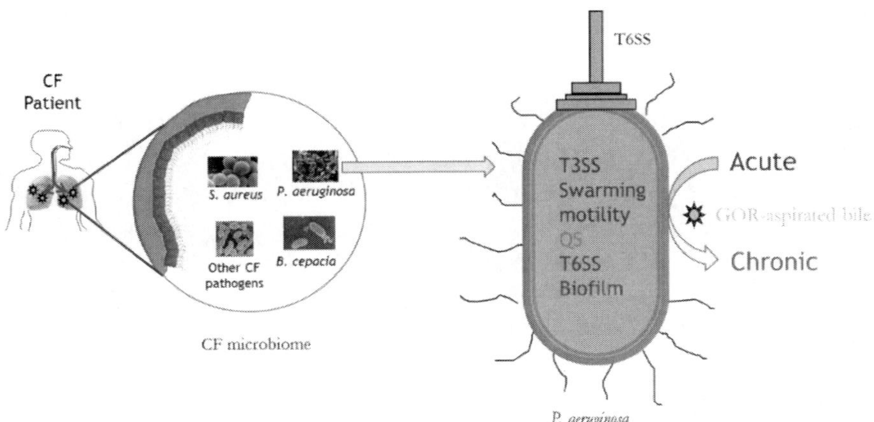

Figure 3. Bile triggers a range of respiratory pathogens particularly *P. aeruginosa* to adopt a chronic biofilm lifestyle through repression of acute virulence systems (shown in red) such as Type three secretion and swarming motility and up regulation of chronic phenotypes (shown in green) such as type six secretion and biofilm production. This aspirated bile also shapes the respiratory microbiome triggering the emergence of these Proteobacterial pathogens.

In severe cases of GORD, where symptoms cannot be controlled by medicinal intervention surgical treatment may be required.

The most common surgery is known as a Nissen fundoplication which involves wrapping the upper curve of the stomach around the oesophagus in an attempt to strengthen the lower oesophageal sphincter muscle which, if successful, prevents recurring reflux. This can be a complete 360 degree wrap or a partial wrap with varying degrees of wrapping (Yates and Oelschlager 2015, Gad El-Hak et al. 2014). This surgery has evolved from an open surgical procedure to a laparoscopic procedure (Yates and Oelschlager 2015, Lv et al. 2015, Dunckley et al. 2014). Additionally, this surgery can now be performed through the mouth avoiding the need for any incisions and is known as a transoral incisionless fundoplication (Reavis and Perry 2014, Rinsma et al. 2014, Witteman et al. 2012). The advantages of surgery are that it addresses the underlying physiological complication of GORD and although it is invasive it is quiet effective in controlling GORD. Patients who undergo this surgery display improvements in lung function which further reinforces that GORD and potentially aspiration of gastric contents into the lungs is contributing to pulmonary decline (Hoppo et al. 2011, Robertson et al. 2012, Hu et al. 2013, Robertson et al. 2010). Endoscopic techniques have been developed and are currently being tested for their effectiveness in the management of GORD. These endoscopic techniques aim at reducing the reliance on long term medication or fundoplication through the creation of a barrier to reflux with very promising results to date. These techniques include radio frequency energy ablation; the most widely utilised technique, endoluminal gastroplasty and numerous implant techniques (Bianco et al. 2006, Dunckley et al. 2014). Radiofrequency ablation also known as the Stretta procedure is one major alternative to surgical intervention. This procedure involves the delivery of consecutive rounds of thermal energy to the lower oesophageal sphincter. Administration is through the use of a 4 channel radio frequency generator and catheter system. As this can be carried out as an outpatient procedure under mild sedation in roughly 35 minutes it would appear an attractive alternative. Though the mechanism of action is still not fully understood it has been shown to be a safe and effective technique for the control of chronic GORD. One potential caveat for its wide scale use is that candidates must be over 18 years of age to qualify for this procedure (Triadafilopoulos 2014, Triadafilopoulos 2003). Endoluminal gastroplasty is a technique developed by Bard Endoscopic technologies which is trademarked as Endocinch. This device uses sutures to create plications in the cardia in an attempt to strengthen the functioning of the LOS.

However this procedure has been associated with complications and moderate side effects such as haemorrhaging, chest pain and dysphagia (Mahmood and Ang 2007, Mahmood et al. 2003). The effectiveness of surgery and endoscopic techniques in controlling GORD suggests that it is aspiration of gastric contents and bile in to the lungs that is possibly responsible for the underlying pathophysiology linking GORD to chronic respiratory disease and not necessarily the effect of acid reflux.

FUTURE PERSPECTIVES

A comprehensive understanding of the behavioural changes induced by bile will facilitate the design of increasingly effective treatment plans for the management of disease. Early intervention is crucial in the long term prevention of bile induced lung damage, with a concerted effort to identify biomarkers for early prognosis. The observation that aspiration status correlated strongly with CF pathophysiology in paediatric patients is highly significant, as bile acid profiling may provide a rapid and effective early prognostic marker for the onset of chronic respiratory infections in these cohorts. Where this is the case, advances in bile acid profiling technologies, possibly to stage where point of care devices are routine in hospitals and clinics, would have significant clinical benefit.

It is clear that bile plays a role in shaping the respiratory microbiome, with individual respiratory pathogens shown to respond to bile by modulating the expression of virulence related signal transduction systems. With the advent of targeted molecular medicine, the identification of sensory pathways involved in the bile induced chronic switch would be a significant advance. This translational research would provide many opportunities for the development of novel therapeutics, which could potentially target the sensory pathways in these respiratory pathogens orchestrating this critical response to bile. Emerging data from a combined transcriptional and functional approach suggest an orchestrated metabolic response to bile that is currently being further explored through metabolomics profiling (Reen et al. 2015 in prep.). Taken together, these molecular insights will provide a pathway with which to decipher and frame the bile response in *P. aeruginosa* and other respiratory pathogens.

The aspiration of bile acids is another example of how the role of bile, and particularly bile acids, in host cellular physiology extends far beyond the classical understanding. With increasing sensitivity, the detection of bile acids at physiologically relevant concentrations, has expanded our appreciation for their role in previously unforeseen circumstances. The next horizon for bile acids research will be deciphering and manipulating their bioactivity for control of the pathophysiology of a range of clinical conditions.

ACKNOWLEDGMENTS

This research was supported in part by grants awarded by the European Commission (FP7-PEOPLE-2013-ITN, 607786; FP7-KBBE-2012-6, CP-TP-312184; FP7-KBBE-2012-6, 311975; OCEAN 2011-2, 287589; Marie Curie 256596; EU-634486), Science Foundation Ireland (SSPC-2, 12/RC/2275; 13/TIDA/B2625; 12/TIDA/B2411; 12/TIDA/B2405; 14/TIDA/2438), the Department of Agriculture and Food (FIRM/RSF/CoFoRD; FIRM 08/RDC/ 629; FIRM 1/F009/MabS; FIRM 13/F/516), the Irish Research Council for Science, Engineering and Technology (PD/2011/2414; GOIPG/2014/647), the Health Research Board/Irish Thoracic Society (MRCG-2014-6), the Marine Institute (Beaufort award C2CRA 2007/082) and Teagasc (Walsh Fellowship 2013).

REFERENCES

Agrawal, A. and Castell, D. 2006. GERD is chronic but not progressive, *J. Clin. Gastroenterol.* 2006 May-Jun;40(5):374-5.

Aguirre, E., Galiana, A., Mira, A., Guardiola, R., Sanchez-Guillen, L., Garcia-Pachon, E., Santibanez, M., Royo, G. and Rodriguez, J. C. 2015. Analysis of microbiota in stable patients with chronic obstructive pulmonary disease. *Apmis*, 123, 427-32.

Aho, V. T., Pereira, P. A., Haahtela, T., Pawankar, R., Auvinen, P. and Koskinen, K. 2015. The microbiome of the human lower airways: a next generation sequencing perspective. *World Allergy Organ J.*, 8, 015-0074.

Akyuz, F., Arici, S., Ermis, F. and Mungan, Z. 2009. Utility of esophageal manometry and pH-metry in gastroesophageal reflux disease before surgery. *Turk. J. Gastroenterol.*, 20, 261-5.

Almagro, P., Salvado, M., Garcia-Vidal, C., Rodriguez-Carballeira, M., Cuchi, E., Torres, J. and Heredia, J. L. 2012. Pseudomonas aeruginosa and mortality after hospital admission for chronic obstructive pulmonary disease. *Respiration,* 84, 36-43.

Altenburg, J., Wortel, K., Van Der Werf, T. S. and Boersma, W. G. 2015. Non-cystic fibrosis bronchiectasis: clinical presentation, diagnosis and treatment, illustrated by data from a Dutch Teaching Hospital. *Neth. J. Med.,* 73, 147-54.

Alvarez-Ortega, C. and Harwood, C. S. 2007. Responses of Pseudomonas aeruginosa to low oxygen indicate that growth in the cystic fibrosis lung is by aerobic respiration. *Molecular microbiology,* 65, 153-165.

Aminov, R. I. A brief history of the antibiotic era: lessons learned and challenges for the future. *Front. Microbiol.,* 1, 2010.

Armougom, F., Bittar, F., Stremler, N., Rolain, J. M., Robert, C., Dubus, J. C., Sarles, J., Raoult, D. and La Scola, B. 2009. Microbial diversity in the sputum of a cystic fibrosis patient studied with 16S rDNA pyrosequencing. *Eur. J. Clin. Microbiol. Infect. Dis.,* 28, 1151-4.

Aseeri, A., Brodlie, M., Lordan, J., Corris, P., Pearson, J., Ward, C. and Manning, N. 2012. Bile acids are present in the lower airways of people with cystic fibrosis, *Am. J. Respir. Crit. Care Med.* 2012 Feb. 15;185(4): 463.

Barnes, P. J. 2011. Glucocorticosteroids: current and future directions. *British Journal of Pharmacology,* 163, 29-43.

Barta, M. L., Guragain, M., Adam, P., Dickenson, N. E., Patil, M., Geisbrecht, B. V., Picking, W. L. and Picking, W. D. 2012. Identification of the bile salt binding site on IpaD from Shigella flexneri and the influence of ligand binding on IpaD structure. *Proteins,* 80, 935-45.

Basler, M., Ho, B. T. and Mekalanos, J. J. 2013. Tit-for-tat: type VI secretion system counterattack during bacterial cell-cell interactions. *Cell,* 152, 884-94.

Beck, J. M., Young, V. B. and Huffnagle, G. B. 2012. The microbiome of the lung. *Transl. Res.,* 160, 258-66.

Begley, M., Gahan, C. G. M. and Hill, C. 2005. The interaction between bacteria and bile. *FEMS Microbiology Reviews,* 29, 625-651.

Berger, G., Bitterman, R. and Azzam, Z. S. 2015. The human microbiota: the rise of an "empire." *Rambam Maimonides Med. J.,* 6.

Bianco, M. A., Rotondano, G., Garofano, M. L. and Cipolletta, L. 2006. Endoscopic treatment of gastro-oesophageal reflux disease. *Acta Otorhinolaryngol. Ital.,* 26, 281-6.

Bittar, F. and Rolain, J. M. 2010. Detection and accurate identification of new or emerging bacteria in cystic fibrosis patients. *Clin. Microbiol. Infect.,* 16, 809-20.

Blainey, P. C., Milla, C. E., Cornfield, D. N. and Quake, S. R. 2012. Quantitative analysis of the human airway microbial ecology reveals a pervasive signature for cystic fibrosis. *Sci. Transl. Med.,* 4.

Bleves, S., Soscia, C., Nogueira-Orlandi, P., Lazdunski, A. and Filloux, A. 2005. Quorum sensing negatively controls type III secretion regulon expression in Pseudomonas aeruginosa PAO1. *J. Bacteriol.,* 187, 3898-902.

Blondeau, K., Dupont, L. J., Mertens, V., Verleden, G., Malfroot, A., Vandenplas, Y., Hauser, B. and Sifrim, D. 2008a. Gastro-oesophageal reflux and aspiration of gastric contents in adult patients with cystic fibrosis. *Gut,* 57, 1049-55.

Blondeau, K., Mertens, V., Vanaudenaerde, B. A., Verleden, G. M., Van Raemdonck, D. E., SIfrim, D. and Dupont, L. J. 2008b. Gastro-oesophageal reflux and gastric aspiration in lung transplant patients with or without chronic rejection. *Eur. Respir. J.,* 31, 707-13.

Blondeau, K., Pauwels, A., Dupont, L., Mertens, V., Proesmans, M., Orel, R., Brecelj, J., Lopez-Alonso, M., Moya, M., Malfroot, A., De WachteR, E., Vandenplas, Y., Hauser, B. and Sifrim, D. 2010. Characteristics of gastroesophageal reflux and potential risk of gastric content aspiration in children with cystic fibrosis. *J. Pediatr. Gastroenterol. Nutr.,* 50, 161-6.

Boutin, S., Graeber, S. Y., Weitnauer, M., Panitz, J., Stahl, M., Clausznitzer, D., Kaderali, L., Einarsson, G., Tunney, M. M., Elborn, J. S., Mall, M. A. and Dalpke, A. H. 2015. Comparison of microbiomes from different niches of upper and lower airways in children and adolescents with cystic fibrosis. *PLoS One,* 10, 2015.

Burkard, I., Von Eckardstein, A. and Rentsch, K. M. 2005. Differentiated quantification of human bile acids in serum by high-performance liquid chromatography-tandem mass spectrometry. *J. Chromatogr. B Analyt. Technol. Biomed. Life Sci.,* 826, 147-59.

Button, B. M., Roberts, S., Kotsimbos, T. C., Levvey, B. J., Williams, T. J., Bailey, M., Snell, G. I. and Wilson, J. W. 2005. Gastroesophageal reflux (symptomatic and silent): a potentially significant problem in patients with cystic fibrosis before and after lung transplantation. *J. Heart Lung Transplant.,* 24, 1522-9.

Carmody, L. A., Zhao, J., Kalikin, L. M., Lebar, W., Simon, R. H., Venkataraman, A., Schmidt, T. M., Abdo, Z., Schloss, P. D. and Lipuma,

J. J. 2015. The daily dynamics of cystic fibrosis airway microbiota during clinical stability and at exacerbation. *Microbiome,* 3, 12.

Carmody, L. A., Zhao, J., Schloss, P. D., Petrosino, J. F., Murray, S., Young, V. B., Li, J. Z. and Lipuma, J. J. 2013. Changes in Cystic Fibrosis Airway Microbiota at Pulmonary Exacerbation. *Annals of the American Thoracic Society,* 10, 179-187.

Charlson, E. S., Bittinger, K., Chen, J., Diamond, J. M., Li, H., Collman, R. G. and Bushman, F. D. 2012a. Assessing bacterial populations in the lung by replicate analysis of samples from the upper and lower respiratory tracts. *PLoS One,* 7, 6.

Charlson, E. S., Bittinger, K., Haas, A. R., Fitzgerald, A. S., Frank, I., Yadav, A., Bushman, F. D. and Collman, R. G. 2011. Topographical continuity of bacterial populations in the healthy human respiratory tract. *Am. J. Respir. Crit. Care Med.,* 184, 957-63.

Charlson, E. S., Diamond, J. M., Bittinger, K., Fitzgerald, A. S., Yadav, A., Haas, A. R., Bushman, F. D. and Collman, R. G. 2012b. Lung-enriched organisms and aberrant bacterial and fungal respiratory microbiota after lung transplant. *Am. J. Respir. Crit. Care Med.,* 186, 536-45.

Choure, A. J., Manali, E. D., Krizmanich, G., Gildea, T. R. and Mehta, A. C. 2005. High Price of Bronchoscopy: Cost of Maintenance and Repair of Flexible Bronchoscopes. *Journal of Bronchology and Interventional Pulmonology,* 12, 147-150.

Coburn, B., Wang, P. W., Diaz Caballero, J., Clark, S. T., Brahma, V., Donaldson, S., Zhang, Y., Surendra, A., Gong, Y., Elizabeth Tullis, D., Yau, Y. C., Waters, V. J., Hwang, D. M. and Guttman, D. S. 2015. Lung microbiota across age and disease stage in cystic fibrosis. *Sci. Rep.,* 5.

Collaco, J. M., Blackman, S. M., Mcgready, J., Naughton, K. M. and Cutting, G. R. 2010. Quantification of the relative contribution of environmental and genetic factors to variation in cystic fibrosis lung function. *J. Pediatr.,* 157, 802-7.

Comito, D., Cascio, A. and Romano, C. 2014. Microbiota biodiversity in inflammatory bowel disease. *Italian Journal of Pediatrics,* 40, 32-32.

Cooper, M. A. and Shlaes, D. 2011. Fix the antibiotics pipeline. *Nature,* 472.

Cox, M. J., Allgaier, M., Taylor, B., Baek, M. S., Huang, Y. J., Daly, R. A., Karaoz, U., Andersen, G. L., Brown, R., Fujimura, K. E., Wu, B., Tran, D., Koff, J., Kleinhenz, M. E., Nielson, D., Brodie, E. L. and Lynch, S. V. 2010. Airway microbiota and pathogen abundance in age-stratified cystic fibrosis patients. *PLoS One,* 5, 0011044.

Cummins, J., Reen, F. J., Baysse, C., Mooij, M. J. and O'Gara, F. 2009. Subinhibitory concentrations of the cationic antimicrobial peptide colistin induce the pseudomonas quinolone signal in Pseudomonas aeruginosa. *Microbiology,* 155, 2826-37.

D'Ovidio, F., Mura, M., Tsang, M., Waddell, T. K., Hutcheon, M. A., Singer, L. G., Hadjiliadis, D., Chaparro, C., Gutierrez, C., Pierre, A., Darling, G., Liu, M. and Keshavjee, S. 2005. Bile acid aspiration and the development of bronchiolitis obliterans after lung transplantation. *J. Thorac. Cardiovasc. Surg.,* 129, 1144-52.

Davies, J. C. 2002. Pseudomonas aeruginosa in cystic fibrosis: pathogenesis and persistence. *Paediatr. Respir. Rev.,* 3, 128-34.

Dean, B. B., Gano, A. D., Jr., Knight, K., Ofman, J. J. and Fass, R. 2004. Effectiveness of proton pump inhibitors in nonerosive reflux disease. *Clin. Gastroenterol. Hepatol.,* 2, 656-64.

Devault, K. R. and Castell, D. O. 2005. Updated guidelines for the diagnosis and treatment of gastroesophageal reflux disease. *Am. J. Gastroenterol.,* 100, 190-200.

Dunckley, M. G., Rajwani, K. M. and Mahomed, A. A. 2014. Laparoscopic watson fundoplication is effective and durable in children with gastrooesophageal reflux. *Minim. Invasive Surg.,* 2014, 409727.

Erb-Downward, J. R. 2012. The Microbiota in Respiratory Disease. *American Journal Of Respiratory And Critical Care Medicine* 185, 1037-1038.

Erb-Downward, J. R., Thompson, D. L., Han, M. K., Freeman, C. M., McCloskey, L., Schmidt, L. A., Young, V. B., Toews, G. B., Curtis, J. L., Sundaram, B., Martinez, F. J. and Huffnagle, G. B. 2011. Analysis of the lung microbiome in the "healthy" smoker and in COPD. *PLoS One,* 6, 0016384.

Feigelson J, S. J. 1975. Gastro-esophagheal reflux in mucoviscidosis. *Nouv. Presse Med.*

Feng, H., Nie, W., Sheoran, A., Zhang, Q. and Tzipori, S. 2006. Bile acids enhance invasiveness of Cryptosporidium spp. into cultured cells. *Infect. Immun.,* 74, 3342-6.

Filkins, L. M., Hampton, T. H., Gifford, A. H., Gross, M. J., Hogan, D. A., Sogin, M. L., Morrison, H. G., Paster, B. J. and O'Toole, G. A. 2012. Prevalence of streptococci and increased polymicrobial diversity associated with cystic fibrosis patient stability. *J. Bacteriol.,* 194, 4709-17.

Flanagan, J. L., Brodie, E. L., Weng, L., Lynch, S. V., Garcia, O., Brown, R., Hugenholtz, P., Desantis, T. Z., Andersen, G. L., Wiener-Kronish, J. P. and Bristow, J. 2007. Loss of bacterial diversity during antibiotic treatment of intubated patients colonized with Pseudomonas aeruginosa. *J. Clin. Microbiol.,* 45, 1954-62.

Flume, P. A., Liou, T. G., Borowitz, D. S., Li, H., Yen, K., Ordoã±ez, C. L., Geller, D. E. and For The, V. X. S. G. 2012. Ivacaftor in Subjects With Cystic Fibrosis Who Are Homozygous for the F508del-CFTR Mutation. *Chest,* 142, 718-724.

Flume, P. A. and Van Devanter, D. R. 2012. State of progress in treating cystic fibrosis respiratory disease. *BMC Medicine,* 10, 88-88.

Frank, D. W. 1997. The exoenzyme S regulon of Pseudomonas aeruginosa. *Mol. Microbiol.,* 26, 621-9.

Gad El-Hak, N., Mostafa, M., Hamdy, E. and Haleem, M. 2014. Short and long-term results of laparoscopic total fundic wrap (Nissen) or semifundoplication (Toupet) for gastroesophageal reflux disease. *Hepatogastroenterology,* 61, 1961-70.

Gaude, G. S. 2009. Pulmonary manifestations of gastroesophageal reflux disease. *Annals of Thoracic Medicine,* 4, 115-123.

Gibson, R. L., Burns, J. L. and Ramsey, B. W. 2003. Pathophysiology and management of pulmonary infections in cystic fibrosis. *Am. J. Respir. Crit. Care Med.,* 168, 918-51.

Goddard, A. F., Staudinger, B. J., Dowd, S. E., Joshi-Datar, A., Wolcott, R. D., Aitken, M. L., Fligner, C. L. and Singh, P. K. 2012. Direct sampling of cystic fibrosis lungs indicates that DNA-based analyses of upper-airway specimens can misrepresent lung microbiota. *Proc. Natl. Acad. Sci. US,* 109, 13769-74.

Gollwitzer, E. S. and Marsland, B. J. 2014. Microbiota abnormalities in inflammatory airway diseases - Potential for therapy. *Pharmacol. Ther.,* 141, 32-9.

Goto, T., Myint, K. T., Sato, K., Wada, O., Kakiyama, G., Iida, T., Hishinuma, T., Mano, N. and Goto, J. 2007. LC/ESI-tandem mass spectrometric determination of bile acid 3-sulfates in human urine 3beta-Sulfooxy-12alpha-hydroxy-5beta-cholanoic acid is an abundant nonamidated sulfate. *J. Chromatogr. B Analyt. Technol. Biomed. Life Sci.,* 846, 69-77.

Gotoh, K., Kodama, T., Hiyoshi, H., Izutsu, K., Park, K. S., Dryselius, R., Akeda, Y., Honda, T. and Iida, T. 2010. Bile acid-induced virulence gene expression of Vibrio parahaemolyticus reveals a novel therapeutic potential for bile acid sequestrants. *PLoS One,* 5, e13365.

Guilbert, T. W. and Denlinger, L. C. 2010. Role of infection in the development and exacerbation of asthma. *Expert Rev. Respir. Med.,* 4, 71-83.

Guina, T., Purvine, S. O., Yo, E. C., Eng, J., Goodlett, D. R., Aebersold, R. and Miller, S. I. 2003. Quantitative proteomic analysis indicates increased synthesis of a quinolone by Pseudomonas aeruginosa isolates from cystic fibrosis airways. *Proc. Natl. Acad. Sci. US,* 100, 2771-6.

Gupta, S. and Chowdhury, R. 1997. Bile affects production of virulence factors and motility of Vibrio cholerae. *Infect. Immun.,* 65, 1131-4.

Guss, A. M., Roeselers, G., Newton, I. L. G., Young, C. R., Klepac-Ceraj, V., Lory, S. and Cavanaugh, C. M. 2011. Phylogenetic and metabolic diversity of bacteria associated with cystic fibrosis. *The ISME journal,* 5, 20-29.

Hajishengallis, G., Darveau, R. P. and Curtis, M. A. 2012. The Keystone Pathogen Hypothesis. *Nature reviews. Microbiology,* 10, 717-725.

Hajishengallis, G., Liang, S., Payne, M. A., Hashim, A., Jotwani, R., Eskan, M. A., McIntosh, M. L., Alsam, A., Kirkwood, K. L., Lambris, J. D., Darveau, R. P. and Curtis, M. A. 2011. A Low-Abundance Biofilm Species Orchestrates Inflammatory Periodontal Disease through the Commensal Microbiota and the Complement Pathway. *Cell host and microbe,* 10, 497-506.

Hallberg, K., Fandriks, L. and Strandvik, B. 2004. Duodenogastric bile reflux is common in cystic fibrosis. *J. Pediatr. Gastroenterol. Nutr.,* 38, 312-6.

Hampton, T. H., Green, D. M., Cutting, G. R., Morrison, H. G., Sogin, M. L., Gifford, A. H., Stanton, B. A. and O'Toole, G. A. 2014. The microbiome in pediatric cystic fibrosis patients: the role of shared environment suggests a window of intervention. *Microbiome,* 2, 2049-2618.

Han, M. K., Huang, Y. J., Lipuma, J. J., Boushey, H. A., Boucher, R. C., Cookson, W. O., Curtis, J. L., Erb-Downward, J., Lynch, S. V., Sethi, S., Toews, G. B., Young, V. B., Wolfgang, M. C., Huffnagle, G. B. and Martinez, F. J. 2012. Significance of the microbiome in obstructive lung disease. *Thorax,* 67, 456-63.

Harris, J. K., De Groote, M. A., Sagel, S. D., Zemanick, E. T., Kapsner, R., Penvari, C., Kaess, H., Deterding, R. R., Accurso, F. J. and Pace, N. R. 2007. Molecular identification of bacteria in bronchoalveolar lavage fluid from children with cystic fibrosis. *Proc. Natl. Acad. Sci. US,* 104, 20529-33.

Hassett, D. J., Borchers, M. T. and Panos, R. J. 2014. Chronic obstructive pulmonary disease (COPD): evaluation from clinical, immunological and bacterial pathogenesis perspectives. *J. Microbiol.,* 52, 211-26.

Hilty, M., Burke, C., Pedro, H., Cardenas, P., Bush, A., Bossley, C., Davies, J., Ervine, A., Poulter, L., Pachter, L., Moffatt, M. F. and Cookson, W. O.

2010. Disordered microbial communities in asthmatic airways. *PLoS One,* 5, 0008578.

Hoiby, N., Bjarnsholt, T., Givskov, M., Molin, S. and Ciofu, O. 2010. Antibiotic resistance of bacterial biofilms. *Int. J. Antimicrob. Agents,* 35, 322-32.

Hoppo, T., Jarido, V., Pennathur, A., Morrell, M., Crespo, M., Shigemura, N., Bermudez, C., Hunter, J. G., Toyoda, Y., Pilewski, J., Luketich, J. D. and Jobe, B. A. 2011. Antireflux surgery preserves lung function in patients with gastroesophageal reflux disease and end-stage lung disease before and after lung transplantation. *Arch. Surg.,* 146, 1041-7.

Hu, Z. W., Wang, Z. G., Zhang, Y., Wu, J. M., Liu, J. J., Lu, F. F., Zhu, G. C. and Liang, W. T. 2013. Gastroesophageal reflux in bronchiectasis and the effect of anti-reflux treatment. *BMC Pulm. Med.,* 13, 34.

Huang, Y. J. and Boushey, H. A. 2015. The microbiome in asthma. *J. Allergy Clin. Immunol.,* 135, 25-30.

Huang, Y. J., Kim, E., Cox, M. J., Brodie, E. L., Brown, R., Wiener-Kronish, J. P. and Lynch, S. V. 2010. A persistent and diverse airway microbiota present during chronic obstructive pulmonary disease exacerbations. *Omics,* 14, 9-59.

Jones, M. L., Martoni, C. J., Ganopolsky, J. G., Labbe, A. and Prakash, S. 2014The human microbiome and bile acid metabolism: dysbiosis, dysmetabolism, disease and intervention. *Expert Opin. Biol. Ther.,* 14, 467-82.

Kakiyama, G., Muto, A., Takei, H., Nittono, H., Murai, T., Kurosawa, T., Hofmann, A. F., Pandak, W. M. and Bajaj, J. S. 2014. A simple and accurate HPLC method for fecal bile acid profile in healthy and cirrhotic subjects: validation by GC-MS and LC-MS. *J. Lipid Res.,* 55, 978-90.

Kanner, R. E., Anthonisen, N. R. and Connett, J. E. 2001. Lower respiratory illnesses promote FEV(1) decline in current smokers but not ex-smokers with mild chronic obstructive pulmonary disease: results from the lung health study. *Am. J. Respir. Crit. Care Med.,* 164, 358-64.

Kapoor, H., Koolwal, A. and Singh, A. 2014. Ivacaftor: A Novel Mutation Modulating Drug. *Journal of Clinical and Diagnostic Research : JCDR,* 8, SE01-SE05.

Khan, T. Z., Wagener, J. S., Bost, T., Martinez, J., Accurso, F. J. and Riches, D. W. 1995. Early pulmonary inflammation in infants with cystic fibrosis. *Am. J. Respir. Crit. Care Med.,* 151, 1075-82.

Korppi, M. 2010. Bacterial infections and pediatric asthma. *Immunol. Allergy Clin. North Am.,* 30, 565-74.

Koskenniemi, K., Laakso, K., Koponen, J., Kankainen, M., Greco, D., Auvinen, P., Savijoki, K., Nyman, T. A., Surakka, A., Salusjarvi, T., De Vos, W. M., Tynkkynen, S., Kalkkinen, N. and Varmanen, P. 2011. Proteomics and transcriptomics characterization of bile stress response in probiotic Lactobacillus rhamnosus GG. *Mol. Cell. Proteomics,* 10, M110. 002741.

Kuczynski, J., Lauber, C. L., Walters, W. A., Parfrey, L. W., Clemente, J. C., Gevers, D. and Knight, R. 2011. Experimental and analytical tools for studying the human microbiome. *Nat. Rev. Genet.,* 13, 47-58.

Lee, A. L., Button, B. M., Denehy, L., Roberts, S., Bamford, T., Mu, F. T., Mifsud, N., Stirling, R. and Wilson, J. W. 2015. Exhaled Breath Condensate Pepsin: Potential Noninvasive Test for Gastroesophageal Reflux in COPD and Bronchiectasis. *Respir. Care,* 60, 244-50.

Lee, T. W., Brownlee, K. G., Conway, S. P., Denton, M. and Littlewood, J. M. 2003. Evaluation of a new definition for chronic Pseudomonas aeruginosa infection in cystic fibrosis patients. *J. Cyst. Fibros.,* 2, 29-34.

Legendre, C., Reen, F. J., Woods, D. F., Mooij, M. J., Adams, C. and O'Gara, F. 2014. Bile acids repress hypoxia-inducible factor 1 signaling and modulate the airway immune response. *Infect. Immun.,* 82, 3531-41.

Levy, S. 2012. Reduced Bacterial Biodiversity Is Associated with Increased Allergy. *Environmental Health Perspectives,* 120, a304-a304.

Lewis, K. 2013. Platforms for antibiotic discovery. *Nat. Rev. Drug Discov.,* 12, 371-87.

Lichtenstein, D. R., Cash, B. D., Davila, R., Baron, T. H., Adler, D. G., Anderson, M. A., Dominitz, J. A., Gan, S. I., Harrison, M. E., 3rd, Ikenberry, S. O., Qureshi, W. A., Rajan, E., Shen, B., Zuckerman, M. J., Fanelli, R. D. and Vanguilder, T. 2007. Role of endoscopy in the management of GERD. *Gastrointest. Endosc.,* 66, 219-24.

Lv, J. M., Huang, D. Y., Lin, H. and Wang, X. F. 2015 [Laparoscopic anti-reflux surgery with biological mesh in treatment of gastroesophageal reflux disease]. *Zhejiang Da Xue Xue Bao Yi Xue Ban,* 44, 74-8.

Lynch, S. V. and Bruce, K. D. 2013. The cystic fibrosis airway microbiome. *Cold Spring Harb. Perspect. Med.,* 3.

Madan, J. C., Koestler, D. C., Stanton, B. A., Davidson, L., Moulton, L. A., Housman, M. L., Moore, J. H., Guill, M. F., Morrison, H. G., Sogin, M. L., Hampton, T. H., Karagas, M. R., Palumbo, P. E., Foster, J. A., Hibberd, P. L. and O'Toole, G. A. 2012. Serial analysis of the gut and respiratory microbiome in cystic fibrosis in infancy: interaction between intestinal and respiratory tracts and impact of nutritional exposures. *MBio*, 3, 00251-12.

Mahenthiralingam, E. 2014. Emerging cystic fibrosis pathogens and the microbiome. *Paediatr. Respir. Rev.*, 1, 13-5.

Mahmood, Z. and Ang, Y. S. 2007. EndoCinch treatment for gastro-oesophageal reflux disease. *Digestion*, 76, 241-7.

Mahmood, Z., McMahon, B. P., Arfin, Q., Byrne, P. J., Reynolds, J. V., Murphy, E. M. and Weir, D. G. 2003. Endocinch therapy for gastro-oesophageal reflux disease: a one year prospective follow up. *Gut*, 52, 34-9.

Main, E., Grillo, L. and Rand, S. 2015. Airway clearance strategies in cystic fibrosis and non-cystic fibrosis bronchiectasis. *Semin. Respir. Crit. Care Med.*, 36, 251-66.

Mano, N., Goto, T., Uchida, M., Nishimura, K., Ando, M., Kobayashi, N. and Goto, J. 2004. Presence of protein-bound unconjugated bile acids in the cytoplasmic fraction of rat brain. *J. Lipid Res.*, 45, 295-300.

Matsui, H., Wagner, V. E., Hill, D. B., Schwab, U. E., Rogers, T. D., Button, B., Taylor, R. M. 2nd, Superfine, R., Rubinstein, M., Iglewski, B. H. and Boucher, R. C. 2006. A physical linkage between cystic fibrosis airway surface dehydration and Pseudomonas aeruginosa biofilms. *Proc. Natl. Acad. Sci. US*, 103, 18131-6.

McDonald, D., Hornig, M., Lozupone, C., Debelius, J., Gilbert, J. A. and Knight, R. 2015. Towards large-cohort comparative studies to define the factors influencing the gut microbial community structure of ASD patients. *Microb. Ecol. Health Dis.*, 26, 2015.

McGowan, J. E., Jr. 2006. Resistance in nonfermenting gram-negative bacteria: multidrug resistance to the maximum. *Am. J. Infect. Control*, 34, S64-73.

Merritt, M. E. and Donaldson, J. R. 2009. Effect of bile salts on the DNA and membrane integrity of enteric bacteria. *J. Med. Microbiol.*, 58, 1533-41.

Mertens, V., Blondeau, K., Pauwels, A., Farre, R., Vanaudenaerde, B., Vos, R., Verleden, G., Van Raemdonck, D. E., Dupont, L. J. and Sifrim, D. 2009. Azithromycin reduces gastroesophageal reflux and aspiration in lung transplant recipients. *Dig. Dis. Sci.*, 54, 972-9.

Mertens, V., Blondeau, K., Van Oudenhove, L., Vanaudenaerde, B., Vos, R., Farre, R., Pauwels, A., Verleden, G., Van Raemdonck, D., Sifrim, D. and Dupont, L. J. 2011. Bile acids aspiration reduces survival in lung transplant recipients with BOS despite azithromycin. *Am. J. Transplant.*, 11, 329-35.

MIllares, L., Ferrari, R., Gallego, M., Garcia-Nuã±ez, M., Pã©rez-Brocal, V., Espasa, M., Pomares, X., Monton, C., Moya, A. and Monsã³, E. 2014. Bronchial microbiome of severe COPD patients colonised by Pseudomonas aeruginosa. *European Journal of Clinical Microbiology and Infectious Diseases,* 33, 1101-1111.

Mougous, J. D., Cuff, M. E., Raunser, S., Shen, A., Zhou, M., Gifford, C. A., Goodman, A. L., Joachimiak, G., Ordonez, C. L., Lory, S., Walz, T., Joachimiak, A. and Mekalanos, J. J. 2006. A virulence locus of Pseudomonas aeruginosa encodes a protein secretion apparatus. *Science,* 312, 1526-30.

Mousa, H. M., Rosen, R., Woodley, F. W., Orsi, M., Armas, D., Faure, C., Fortunato, J., O'Connor, J., Skaggs, B. and Nurko, S. 2011. Esophageal Impedance Monitoring for Gastroesophageal Reflux. *Journal of Pediatric Gastroenterology and Nutrition,* 52, 129-139 10.1097/MPG.0b013e3181 ffde67.

Mussaffi, H., Fireman, E. M., Mei-Zahav, M., Prais, D. and Blau, H. 2008. Induced sputum in the very young: a new key to infection and inflammation. *Chest,* 133, 176-82.

Nagalingam, N. A., Cope, E. K. and Lynch, S. V. 2013. Probiotic strategies for treatment of respiratory diseases. *Trends Microbiol.,* 21, 485-92.

Neujahr, D. C., Uppal, K., Force, S. D., Fernandez, F., Lawrence, C., Pickens, A., Bag, R., Lockard, C., Kirk, A. D., Tran, V., Lee, K., Jones, D. P. and Park, Y. 2014. Bile acid aspiration associated with lung chemical profile linked to other biomarkers of injury after lung transplantation. *Am. J. Transplant.,* 14, 841-8.

Nichols, D., Chmiel, J. and Berger, M. 2008. Chronic inflammation in the cystic fibrosis lung: alterations in inter- and intracellular signaling. *Clin. Rev. Allergy Immunol.,* 34, 146-62.

NIU 2014. Characterization of Bile Acids and Its Application in Quality Control of Cow-Bezoar and Bear Bile Powder.

O'Callaghan, J., Reen, F. J., Adams, C., Casey, P. G., Gahan, C. G. and O'Gara, F. 2012. A novel host-responsive sensor mediates virulence and type III secretion during Pseudomonas aeruginosa-host cell interactions. *Microbiology,* 158, 1057-70.

O'Callaghan, J., Reen, F. J., Adams, C. and O'Gara, F. 2011. Low oxygen induces the type III secretion system in Pseudomonas aeruginosa via modulation of the small RNAs rsmZ and rsmY. *Microbiology,* 157, 3417-28.

Olive, A. J., Kenjale, R., Espina, M., Moore, D. S., Picking, W. L. and Picking, W. D. 2007. Bile salts stimulate recruitment of IpaB to the Shigella flexneri surface, where it colocalizes with IpaD at the tip of the type III secretion needle. *Infect. Immun.*, 75, 2626-9.

Papi, A., Bellettato, C. M., Braccioni, F., Romagnoli, M., Casolari, P., Caramori, G., Fabbri, L. M. and Johnston, S. L. 2006. Infections and airway inflammation in chronic obstructive pulmonary disease severe exacerbations. *Am. J. Respir. Crit. Care Med.*, 173, 1114-21.

Parkins, M. D., Sibley, C. D., Surette, M. G. and Rabin, H. R. 2008. The Streptococcus milleri group--an unrecognized cause of disease in cystic fibrosis: a case series and literature review. *Pediatr. Pulmonol.*, 43, 490-7.

Patel, A. K., Singhania, R. R., Pandey, A. and Chincholkar, S. B. 2010. Probiotic bile salt hydrolase: current developments and perspectives. *Appl. Biochem. Biotechnol.*, 162, 166-80.

Patrick, L. 2011. Gastroesophageal reflux disease (GERD): a review of conventional and alternative treatments. *Altern. Med. Rev.*, 16, 116-33.

Pauwels, A., Decraene, A., Blondeau, K., Mertens, V., Farre, R., Proesmans, M., Van Bleyenbergh, P., Sifrim, D. and Dupont, L. J. 2012. Bile acids in sputum and increased airway inflammation in patients with cystic fibrosis. *Chest,* 141, 1568-74.

Perwaiz, S., Tuchweber, B., Mignault, D., Gilat, T. and Yousef, I. M. 2001. Determination of bile acids in biological fluids by liquid chromatography-electrospray tandem mass spectrometry. *J. Lipid Res.*, 42, 114-9.

Potvin, E., Lehoux, D. E., Kukavica-Ibrulj, I., Richard, K. L., Sanschagrin, F., Lau, G. W. and Levesque, R. C. 2003. In vivo functional genomics of Pseudomonas aeruginosa for high-throughput screening of new virulence factors and antibacterial targets. *Environ. Microbiol.*, 5, 1294-308.

Pragman, A. A., Kim, H. B., Reilly, C. S., Wendt, C. and Isaacson, R. E. 2012. The lung microbiome in moderate and severe chronic obstructive pulmonary disease. *PLoS One,* 7, 11.

Pressler, T., Bohmova, C., Conway, S., Dumcius, S., Hjelte, L., Hoiby, N., Kollberg, H., Tummler, B. and Vavrova, V. 2011. Chronic Pseudomonas aeruginosa infection definition: EuroCareCF Working Group report. *J. Cyst. Fibros.*, 2011, 60011-8.

Proctor, L. M. 2011. The Human Microbiome Project in 2011 and beyond. *Cell Host Microbe,* 10, 287-91.

Prouty, A. M., Brodsky, I. E., Manos, J., Belas, R., Falkow, S. and Gunn, J. S. 2004. Transcriptional regulation of Salmonella enterica serovar

Typhimurium genes by bile. *FEMS Immunol. Med. Microbiol.,* 41, 177-85.

Prouty, A. M. and Gunn, J. S. 2000. Salmonella enterica serovar typhimurium invasion is repressed in the presence of bile. *Infect. Immun.,* 68, 6763-9.

Quillin, S. J., Schwartz, K. T. and Leber, J. H. 2011. The novel Listeria monocytogenes bile sensor BrtA controls expression of the cholic acid efflux pump MdrT. *Mol. Microbiol.,* 81, 129-42.

Rackoff, A., Agrawal, A., Hila, A., Mainie, I., Tutuian, R. and Castell, D. O. 2005. Histamine-2 receptor antagonists at night improve gastroesophageal reflux disease symptoms for patients on proton pump inhibitor therapy. *Dis. Esophagus,* 18, 370-3.

Rao, S. and Grigg, J. 2006. New insights into pulmonary inflammation in cystic fibrosis. *Arch. Dis. Child,* 91, 786-8.

Reavis, K. M. and Perry, K. A. 2014. Transoral incisionless fundoplication for the treatment of gastroesophageal reflux disease. *Expert Rev. Med. Devices,* 11, 341-50.

Reder, N. P., Davis, C. S., Kovacs, E. J. and Fisichella, P. M. 2014. The diagnostic value of gastroesophageal reflux disease (GERD) symptoms and detection of pepsin and bile acids in bronchoalveolar lavage fluid and exhaled breath condensate for identifying lung transplantation patients with GERD-induced aspiration. *Surg. Endosc.,* 28, 1794-800.

Redinbo, M. R. 2014. The microbiota, chemical symbiosis, and human disease. *J. Mol. Biol.,* 426, 3877-91.

Reen, F. J., Barret, M., Fargier, E., O'Muinneachain, M. and O'Gara, F. 2013. Molecular evolution of LysR-type transcriptional regulation in Pseudomonas aeruginosa. *Mol. Phylogenet. Evol.,* 66, 1041-9.

Reen, F. J., Mooij, M. J., Holcombe, L. J., McSweeney, C. M., McGlacken, G. P., Morrissey, J. P. and O'Gara, F. 2011. The Pseudomonas quinolone signal (PQS), and its precursor HHQ, modulate interspecies and interkingdom behaviour. *FEMS Microbiol. Ecol.,* 77, 413-28.

Reen, F. J., Shanahan, R., Cano, R., O'Gara, F. and McGlacken, G. P. 2015. A structure activity-relationship study of the bacterial signal molecule HHQ reveals swarming motility inhibition in Bacillus atrophaeus. *Org. Biomol. Chem.,* 13, 5537-41.

Reen, F. J., Woods, D. F., Mooij, M. J., Adams, C. and O'GARA, F. 2012. Respiratory pathogens adopt a chronic lifestyle in response to bile. *PLoS One,* 7, 26.

Reen, F. J., Woods, D. F., Mooij, M. J., Chroinin, M. N., Mullane, D., Zhou, L., Quille, J., Fitzpatrick, D., Glennon, J. D., McGlacken, G. P., Adams,

C. and O'Gara, F. 2014. Aspirated bile: a major host trigger modulating respiratory pathogen colonisation in cystic fibrosis patients. *Eur. J. Clin. Microbiol. Infect. Dis.,* 33, 1763-71.

Renwick, J., McNally, P., John, B., Desantis, T., Linnane, B., Murphy, P. and on behalf of, S. C. 2014. The Microbial Community of the Cystic Fibrosis Airway Is Disrupted in Early Life. *PLoS One,* 9, e109798.

Rinsma, N. F., Smeets, F. G., Bruls, D. W., Kessing, B. F., Bouvy, N. D., masclee, A. A. and Conchillo, J. M. 2014. Effect of transoral incisionless fundoplication on reflux mechanisms. *Surg. Endosc.,* 28, 941-9.

Roberts, S. and Thornington, R. E. 2005. Paediatric bronchoscopy. *Continuing Education in Anaesthesia, Critical Care and Pain,* 5.

Robertson, A. G., Krishnan, A., Ward, C., Pearson, J. P., Small, T., Corris, P. A., Dark, J. H., Karat, D., Shenfine, J. and Griffin, S. M. 2012. Anti-reflux surgery in lung transplant recipients: outcomes and effects on quality of life. *Eur. Respir. J.,* 39, 691-7.

Robertson, A. G., Ward, C., Pearson, J. P., Corris, P. A., Dark, J. H. and Griffin, S. M. 2010. Lung transplantation, gastroesophageal reflux, and fundoplication. *Ann. Thorac. Surg.,* 89, 653-60.

Roda, A., Gioacchini, A. M., Cerre, C. and Baraldini, M. 1995. High-performance liquid chromatographic-electrospray mass spectrometric analysis of bile acids in biological fluids. *J. Chromatogr. B Biomed. Appl.,* 665, 281-94.

Rogers, G. B., Carroll, M. P., Serisier, D. J., Hockey, P. M., Jones, G. and Bruce, K. D. 2004. Characterization of Bacterial Community Diversity in Cystic Fibrosis Lung Infections by Use of 16S Ribosomal DNA Terminal Restriction Fragment Length Polymorphism Profiling. *Journal of Clinical Microbiology,* 42, 5176-5183.

Rogers, G. B., Carroll, M. P., Serisier, D. J., Hockey, P. M., Jones, G., Kehagia, V., Connett, G. J. and Bruce, K. D. 2006. Use of 16S rRNA gene profiling by terminal restriction fragment length polymorphism analysis to compare bacterial communities in sputum and mouthwash samples from patients with cystic fibrosis. *J. Clin. Microbiol.,* 44, 2601-4.

Samareh fekri, M., Poursalehi, H. R., Najafipour, H., Dabiri, S., Shokoohi, M., Siahposht Khacheki, A., Shahrokhi, N., Malekpour Afshar, R. and Lashkarizadeh, M. R. 2013. Pulmonary Complications of Gastric Fluid and Bile Salts Aspiration, an Experimental Study in Rat. *Iranian Journal of Basic Medical Sciences,* 16, 790-796.

Schadt, E. E., Turner, S. and Kasarskis, A. 2010. A window into third-generation sequencing. *Hum. Mol. Genet.,* 19, 21.

Schultz, A. and Stick, S. 2015. Early pulmonary inflammation and lung damage in children with cystic fibrosis. *Respirology,* 20, 569-78.

Scott, M. and Gelhot, A. R. 1999. Gastroesophageal reflux disease: diagnosis and management. *Am. Fam. Physician,* 59, 1161-9.

Sethi, S., Mallia, P. and Johnston, S. L. 2009. New paradigms in the pathogenesis of chronic obstructive pulmonary disease II. *Proc. Am. Thorac. Soc.,* 6, 532-4.

Sibley, C. D., Grinwis, M. E., Field, T. R., Eshaghurshan, C. S., Faria, M. M., Dowd, S. E., Parkins, M. D., Rabin, H. R. and Surette, M. G. 2011. Culture enriched molecular profiling of the cystic fibrosis airway microbiome. *PLoS One,* 6, 28.

Sibley, C. D., Parkins, M. D., Rabin, H. R., Duan, K., Norgaard, J. C. and Surette, M. G. 2008. A polymicrobial perspective of pulmonary infections exposes an enigmatic pathogen in cystic fibrosis patients. *Proc. Natl. Acad. Sci. US,* 105, 15070-5.

Sibley, C. D., Rabin, H. and Surette, M. G. 2006. Cystic fibrosis: a polymicrobial infectious disease. *Future Microbiol.,* 1, 53-61.

Singh, P. K., Schaefer, A. L., Parsek, M. R., Moninger, T. O., Welsh, M. J. and Greenberg, E. P. 2000. Quorum-sensing signals indicate that cystic fibrosis lungs are infected with bacterial biofilms. *Nature,* 407, 762-4.

Sontag, S. J., Sonnenberg, A., Schnell, T. G., Leya, J. and Metz, A. 2006. The long-term natural history of gastroesophageal reflux disease. *J. Clin. Gastroenterol.,* 40, 398-404.

Staley, J. T. and Konopka, A. 1985. Measurement of in situ activities of nonphotosynthetic microorganisms in aquatic and terrestrial habitats. *Annu. Rev. Microbiol.,* 39, 321-46.

Staudinger, B. J., Muller, J. F., Halldorsson, S., Boles, B., Angermeyer, A., Nguyen, D., Rosen, H., Baldursson, O., Gottfreethsson, M., Guethmundsson, G. H. and SINGH, P. K. 2014. Conditions associated with the cystic fibrosis defect promote chronic Pseudomonas aeruginosa infection. *Am. J. Respir. Crit. Care Med.,* 189, 812-24.

Stokell, J. R., Gharaibeh, R. Z., Hamp, T. J., Zapata, M. J., Fodor, A. A. and Steck, T. R. 2015. Analysis of Changes in Diversity and Abundance of the Microbial Community in a Cystic Fibrosis Patient over a Multiyear Period. *Journal of Clinical Microbiology,* 53, 237-247.

Stressmann, F. A., Rogers, G. B., Klem, E. R., Lilley, A. K., Donaldson, S. H., Daniels, T. W., Carroll, M. P., Patel, N., Forbes, B., Boucher, R. C., Wolfgang, M. C. and Bruce, K. D. 2011. Analysis of the bacterial communities present in lungs of patients with cystic fibrosis from American and British centers. *J. Clin. Microbiol.,* 49, 281-91.

Surette, M. G. 2014. The cystic fibrosis lung microbiome. *Ann. Am. Thorac. Soc.,* 2014, 201306-159MG.

Sweet, M. P., Patti, M. G., Hoopes, C., Hays, S. R. and Golden, J. A. 2009. Gastro-oesophageal reflux and aspiration in patients with advanced lung disease. *Thorax,* 64, 167-73.

Sze, M. A., Dimitriu, P. A., Hayashi, S., Elliott, W. M., McDonough, J. E., Gosselink, J. V., Cooper, J., Sin, D. D., Mohn, W. W. and Hogg, J. C. 2012. The lung tissue microbiome in chronic obstructive pulmonary disease. *Am. J. Respir. Crit. Care Med.,* 185, 1073-80.

Thomson, A. B. R. 2008. Impact of PPIs on patient focused symptomatology in GERD. *Therapeutics and Clinical Risk Management,* 4, 1185-1200.

Triadafilopoulos, G. 2003. Stretta: an effective, minimally invasive treatment for gastroesophageal reflux disease. *Am. J. Med.,* 115 Suppl. 3A, 192s-200s.

Triadafilopoulos, G. 2014. The great beyond: radiofrequency ablation for hemostasis. *Endoscopy,* 46, 925-6.

Tunney, M. M., Field, T. R., Moriarty, T. F., Patrick, S., Doering, G., Muhlebach, M. S., Wolfgang, M. C., boucher, R., Gilpin, D. F., McDowell, A. and Elborn, J. S. 2008. Detection of anaerobic bacteria in high numbers in sputum from patients with cystic fibrosis. *Am. J. Respir. Crit. Care Med.,* 177, 995-1001.

Twigg, H. L., 3rd, Morris, A., Ghedin, E., Curtis, J. L., Huffnagle, G. B., Crothers, K., Campbell, T. B., Flores, S. C., Fontenot, A. P., Beck, J. M., Huang, L., Lynch, S., Knox, K. S. and Weinstock, G. 2013. Use of bronchoalveolar lavage to assess the respiratory microbiome: signal in the noise. *Lancet Respir. Med.,* 1, 354-6.

Ursell, L. K., Metcalf, J. L., Parfrey, L. W. and Knight, R. 2012. Defining the human microbiome. *Nutr. Rev.,* 2012, 1753-4887.

Vakil, N., Van Zanten, S. V., Kahrilas, P., Dent, J. and Jones, R. 2006. The Montreal definition and classification of gastroesophageal reflux disease: a global evidence-based consensus. *Am. J. Gastroenterol.,* 101, 1900-20.

Vallis, A. J., Finck-Barbancon, V., Yahr, T. L. and Frank, D. W. 1999. Biological effects of Pseudomonas aeruginosa type III-secreted proteins on CHO cells. *Infect. Immun.,* 67, 2040-4.

Vestbo, J., Prescott, E. and Lange, P. 1996. Association of chronic mucus hypersecretion with FEV1 decline and chronic obstructive pulmonary disease morbidity. Copenhagen City Heart Study Group. *Am. J. Respir. Crit. Care Med.,* 153, 1530-5.

Wainwright, C. E., Elborn, J. S., Ramsey, B. W., Marigowda, G., Huang, X., cipolli, M., Colombo, C., Davies, J. C., De Boeck, K., Flume, P. A., Konstan, M. W., McColley, S. A., McCoy, K., McKone, E. F., Munck, A., Ratjen, F., Rowe, S. M., Waltz, D. and Boyle, M. P. 2015. Lumacaftor-Ivacaftor in Patients with Cystic Fibrosis Homozygous for Phe508del CFTR. *New England Journal of Medicine,* 373, 220-231.

Weiner, J. R., Toy, E. L., Sacco, P. and Duh, M. S. 2008. Costs, quality of life and treatment compliance associated with antibiotic therapies in patients with cystic fibrosis: a review of the literature. *Expert Opin. Pharmacother.,* 9, 751-66.

Willner, D., Haynes, M. R., Furlan, M., Schmieder, R., Lim, Y. W., Rainey, P. B., Rohwer, F. and Conrad, D. 2012. Spatial distribution of microbial communities in the cystic fibrosis lung. *Isme J.,* 6, 471-4.

Witteman, B. P., Strijkers, R., De Vries, E., Toemen, L., Conchillo, J. M., Hameeteman, W., Dagnelie, P. C., Koek, G. H. and Bouvy, N. D. 2012. Transoral incisionless fundoplication for treatment of gastroesophageal reflux disease in clinical practice. *Surg. Endosc.,* 26, 3307-15.

Worlitzsch, D., Tarran, R., Ulrich, M., Schwab, U., Cekici, A., Meyer, K. C., Birrer, P., Bellon, G., Berger, J., Weiss, T., Botzenhart, K., Yankaskas, J. R., Randell, S., Boucher, R. C. and Doring, G. 2002. Effects of reduced mucus oxygen concentration in airway Pseudomonas infections of cystic fibrosis patients. *J. Clin. Invest.,* 109, 317-25.

Wu, Y. C., Hsu, P. K., Su, K. C., Liu, L. Y., Tsai, C. C., Tsai, S. H., Hsu, W. H., Lee, Y. C. and Perng, D. W. 2009. Bile acid aspiration in suspected ventilator-associated pneumonia. *Chest,* 136, 118-24.

Yang, L., Nilsson, M., Gjermansen, M., Givskov, M. and Tolker-Nielsen, T. 2009. Pyoverdine and PQS mediated subpopulation interactions involved in Pseudomonas aeruginosa biofilm formation. *Mol. Microbiol.,* 74, 1380-92.

YateS, R. B. and Oelschlager, B. K. 2015. Surgical treatment of gastroesophageal reflux disease. *Surg. Clin. North Am.,* 95, 527-53.

Zemanick, E. T., Sagel, S. D. and Harris, J. K. 2011. The airway microbiome in cystic fibrosis and implications for treatment. *Curr. Opin. Pediatr.,* 23, 319-24.

INDEX

A

acetylcholine, 7, 14
acidic, 3
active compound, 17
acute infection, ix, 58
adaptation, 78
adenine, 73
adhesion, 14
adipose, 7, 8
adipose tissue, 7, 8
adolescents, 84
adsorption, 23
adults, 64
advancements, 73
aerobic bacteria, 67
age, 10, 68, 80, 85
aggregation, 25, 26, 27, 29, 30, 50, 51, 54
aggregation process, 50
airway inflammation, 62, 93
airway remodelling, 61
airways, 61, 64, 74, 82, 83, 84, 88
alternative treatments, 93
alters, 4
amino, 42
amphiphiles, 17, 18
anaerobic bacteria, 67, 97
antibiotic, ix, 58, 62, 69, 72, 76, 83, 86, 90, 98
antibiotic resistance, 62

apoptosis, 4, 11, 12
aqueous solutions, 51, 53
aspiration, vii, viii, 57, 58, 60, 72, 73, 74, 76, 80, 81, 84, 86, 91, 92, 94, 97, 98
asthma, viii, 57, 59, 62, 66, 70, 74, 87, 89
asthmatic airways, 89
asymptomatic, 71
atherosclerosis, 4, 10, 14
atoms, 30, 47, 48
ATP, 39, 53, 60
autosomal recessive, 60

B

bacteria, ix, 58, 62, 63, 65, 66, 67, 68, 69, 76, 83, 84, 88, 91
barriers, viii, 18, 71
Beijing, 1
bile acid receptors, vii, 1, 2
bile acid sequestrant, vii, viii, 2, 7, 87
bile acids, vii, viii, 1, 2, 3, 6, 10, 11, 13, 15, 17, 19, 23, 24, 29, 30, 31, 32, 35, 39, 41, 47, 49, 50, 54, 55, 57, 72, 73, 76, 81, 84, 91, 93, 94, 95
bile aspiration, 57, 72
bilirubin, 32
biochemistry, 46
biodiversity, ix, 58, 61, 74, 75, 85
biological fluids, 93, 95
biomarkers, 72, 81, 92

biomolecules, 32
biosynthesis, 3, 5
blood, 73
Boltzmann constant, 44
bonding, 18, 52
bonds, 19, 20, 29, 30, 32
BOS, 91
brain, 73, 91
breathlessness, 62
bronchial asthma, 70
bronchiectasis, 59, 62, 66, 83, 89, 91
bronchiolitis, 72, 73, 86
bronchiolitis obliterans syndrome, 72, 73
bronchitis, 70
bronchoscopy, 64, 95

C

cancer, viii, 2, 5, 6, 7, 8, 9, 11, 14, 15
cancer cells, 11, 15
candidates, 80
carbohydrate, 13
carbohydrate metabolism, 13
carbon atoms, 19, 30
carboxyl, 3, 27
carboxyle, 32
carcinogenesis, 15
catabolism, 3
catheter, 72, 80
cation, 30
Caucasian population, 60
cell line, 8, 15
cell signaling, 2, 4, 5, 6
challenges, 83
chemical, viii, 8, 17, 42, 53, 92, 94
chemical bonds, 42
childhood, 76
children, 84, 86, 88, 96
China, 1, 9
Chlamydia, 62
CHO cells, 97
cholangiocarcinoma, 7, 11, 14
cholanoic, 19, 20, 21, 25, 29, 31, 46, 87
cholecystectomy, 11
cholera, 76
cholestasis, 4, 12, 54
cholesterol, vii, viii, 1, 2, 3, 4, 17, 31, 32, 38, 39, 42, 52, 53
cholic acid, 3, 24, 25, 26, 27, 28, 31, 33, 38, 46, 52, 94
choline, 33
chromatography, 23, 50, 73
Chronic Lifestyle, 75
chronic obstructive pulmonary disease (COPD), viii, 57, 59, 60, 61, 66, 69, 70, 71, 74, 82, 83, 86, 88, 89, 92, 93, 96, 97, 98
chronic rejection, 84
chronic respiratory diseases, 59
chronic respiratory infection, vii, 73, 81
circulation, 5, 12
classification, 61, 97
clinical diagnosis, 71
clinical presentation, 83
clinical symptoms, 61, 71
coenzyme, 73
colon, 3, 15, 19
colonisation, 72, 95
colorectal cancer, 9
communication, 78
communities, 63, 65, 66, 68, 69, 70, 95, 97
community, ix, 58, 66, 68
complement, 3
complexity, 65, 74
compliance, 98
complications, 81
composition, 43, 49, 67, 69
compounds, 9, 19, 55
computer, 51
conductivity, 31, 32
configuration, 42, 44
conjugation, 3, 5
consensus, 97
contamination, 64, 65
control group, 70
controversial, 67
correlation, 46, 67, 69, 70, 72, 74, 75
corticosteroids, 62
cost, 59
cough, 70

coughing, 64
critical micelle concentration (CMC), 18, 25, 26, 30, 39, 40, 46, 47, 48, 50
cross sectional study, 68
crystalline, 40, 52
culture, 65, 68, 72
cyclooxygenase, 7, 11
cystic fibrosis (CF), viii, 57, 58, 59, 60, 61, 62, 65, 66, 67, 68, 69, 70, 71, 72, 73, 74, 75, 76, 78, 81, 83, 84, 85, 86, 87, 88, 89, 90, 91, 92, 93, 94, 95, 96, 97, 98
cytochrome, 3
cytoplasm, 6, 39

D

DCA, 3, 9
defects, 10
dehydration, 91
delayed gastric emptying, 71
Department of Agriculture, 82
deprivation, 11
derivatives, vii, viii, 2, 3, 18, 19, 25, 30, 31, 46, 47, 49, 50, 51, 55
destruction, 46, 62, 67
detection, 65, 71, 72, 73, 81, 94
detergents, 38
detoxification, 5
deviation, 43
diabetes, viii, 4, 5, 7, 15, 57, 75
diet, 9
diffraction, 36
diffusion, 39, 67
digestion, viii, 9, 17
dilation, 61
disability, 59
disease progression, ix, 58, 59, 61, 62, 63, 69, 70
diseases, vii, viii, 2, 4, 5, 6, 7, 9, 10, 57, 59, 62, 63, 75, 76, 87, 92
distribution, 24, 28, 40, 43, 54, 98
diversity, 66, 68, 69, 78, 83, 86, 88
DNA, 6, 65, 66, 87, 91, 95
drugs, viii, 18, 32, 46, 72
dysphagia, 81

E

ecology, 84
electrolyte, 50
electron, 54
electron microscopy, 54
encoding, 60
endocrine, 4, 7
endoscopy, 71, 90
endothelial cells, 14
energy, vii, viii, 2, 5, 8, 9, 13, 18, 23, 29, 42, 43, 44, 45, 46, 80
energy expenditure, 8, 13
entropy, 18, 23, 32, 42, 43, 44
environment(s), viii, 18, 22, 23, 28, 32, 39, 60, 63, 64, 65, 66, 67, 69, 88
environmental factors, 67
enzimatically, 19
enzyme(s), 3, 5, 6, 7, 8, 73
eosinophil, 62
epithelial cells, 72
epithelium, 64
equilibrium, 30, 52
ERS, 59, 62
ESI, 87
esophagitis, 71
ethanol, 32
European Commission, 82
European Union, 59
evidence, ix, 49, 53, 54, 58, 68, 69, 71, 72, 74, 97
evolution, 30, 68, 94
Excess Gibbs energy, 29, 43
exclusion, 53
experimental design, 70
exporter(s), 39
exposure, 9, 78
extraction, 66

F

farnesoid X receptor (FXR), vii, 1, 2, 2, 4, 5, 7, 8, 9, 10, 11, 12, 13, 39
fasting, 11

fat, vii, 1, 2
fatty acid(s), vii, viii, 2, 6, 33, 54
fibrinogen, 13
fibroblast growth factor, 11
fibroblasts, 7, 14
fibrosis, 59, 61, 62, 70, 91, 96
flora, 3
fluctuations, 73
fluid, 59, 63, 64, 88, 94
force, 29, 49
formation, ix, 18, 26, 27, 29, 30, 31, 38, 40,
    41, 42, 43, 45, 48, 49, 51, 52, 53, 54, 58,
    77, 78, 98
formula, 21, 23, 30, 47
freedom, 18
functional approach, 81

G

gallbladder, viii, 17
gastroenteritis, 76
gastroesophageal reflux, 82, 84, 86, 87, 89,
    90, 91, 94, 95, 96, 97, 98
gastro-oesophageal reflux disease, 70, 83,
    91
gene expression, 6, 7, 8, 13, 87
genes, 4, 5, 94
genetic disease, 60
genetic factors, 85
genomics, 93
Gibbs energy, 29, 42, 43, 45, 46
glucagon, 8, 14
gluconeogenesis, 6, 7
glucose, vii, viii, 2, 4, 5, 6, 7, 8, 9, 15
glycine, 3
Gpbar1, vii, 1, 2, 4, 11, 14
G-protein-coupled bile acid receptor, vii, 1,
    2, 11, 14
grants, 82
growth, 4, 7, 9, 14, 53, 68, 76, 78, 83
guidelines, 86

H

habitats, 96
health, 7, 10, 59, 66, 89
heartburn, 71
height, 35
hemolytic potential, 46, 47, 48
hemostasis, 97
hepatocarcinogenesis, 4
hepatocellular carcinoma, 9, 11
hepatocytes, viii, 17, 41
heterogeneity, 68
high fat, 9
history, 83, 96
homeostasis, 5, 7, 9, 12, 13
hormone, vii, 1, 2, 4, 8, 13
host, vii, ix, 58, 63, 69, 70, 74, 77, 78, 81,
    88, 92, 95
human, 3, 5, 7, 8, 12, 15, 53, 65, 73, 76, 82,
    83, 84, 85, 87, 89, 90, 94, 97
Hunter, 89
hydrogen, 18, 20, 21, 22, 23, 29, 31, 32, 38,
    44, 52
hydrogen atoms, 20
hydrogen bonds, 18, 21, 22, 23, 29, 31, 32,
    38
hydrophobicity, 18, 23, 24, 29, 47, 49, 50,
    54
hydroxyl, 21, 23, 24, 27, 28, 47, 73
hydroxyl groups, 24, 28
hyperglycemia, 7
hypertonic saline, 64
hypoglycemia, 7
hypothesis, 59, 66, 72, 78
hypoxia, 90
hypoxia-inducible factor, 90

I

ideal, 43
identification, 65, 66, 73, 76, 81, 84, 88
idiopathic, 59, 62
ileum, 3
immune response, 60, 90

immune system, 59, 61
improvements, 80
in vitro, 11, 46
in vivo, 11
incidence, 9, 71, 72
individuals, ix, 58, 62, 63, 67
induction, 5, 8, 9
industry, 63
infancy, 90
infants, 89
infection, vii, ix, 58, 59, 60, 61, 67, 68, 70,
    73, 76, 77, 87, 90, 92, 93, 96
inflammation, viii, 2, 5, 9, 10, 14, 59, 60,
    61, 62, 70, 72, 89, 92, 94, 96
inflammatory bowel disease, 85
inflammatory disease, 62
influenza a, 67
inhibition, 94
inhibitor, 71, 79, 94
initial state, 38
injury, 4, 7, 9, 92
insulin, 7, 8
insulin sensitivity, 7
integrity, 47, 91
intervention, 69, 80, 81, 88, 89
intestinal flora, 19
intestine, 4, 5, 12
ionization, 73
Ireland, 57, 82

L

Lactobacillus, 90
LC-MS, 73, 89
lecithin, 32, 33, 34, 35, 36, 37, 38, 39, 40,
    41, 42, 43, 47, 48, 52, 53, 54
lesions, 8
life expectancy, 62
ligand, 6, 83
light, 11, 53, 70, 78
light scattering, 53
linear congeneric groups, 29
linear dependence, 36
lipid metabolism, 4, 5, 9
lipids, vii, viii, 1, 2, 17, 54

lipoprotein(s), vii, viii, 2, 5, 6, 13
liquid chromatography, 53, 73, 84, 93
liquid crystal phase, 36
liquid crystals, 36
liquid phase, 41
Listeria monocytogenes, 76, 94
liver, viii, 2, 3, 4, 5, 6, 9, 10, 14, 15, 17, 19,
    39, 45, 48, 53, 54
liver cells, 10
local community, 69
localization, 14
locus, 92
lumen, 39, 41, 45, 49
lung disease, ix, 58, 60, 65, 72, 73, 89, 97
lung function, ix, 58, 59, 60, 61, 66, 68, 69,
    72, 80, 85, 89
Lung Microbiome, 63
lung transplantation, 62, 64, 65, 72, 84, 86,
    89, 92, 94

M

macrophages, 6
majority, 65, 67, 79
mammals, 3
management, ix, 58, 59, 62, 67, 76, 77, 79,
    80, 81, 87, 90, 96
manipulation, 67
mantle, 34
mass, 8, 34, 73, 84, 87, 93, 95
mass spectrometry, 73, 84, 93
matter, 49
measurement(s), 32, 68
media, 40
median, 76
medical, 67
medication, 80
membrane permeability, viii, 18
membranes, 54
messenger RNA, 7
metabolic, 10
metabolic disorder(s), vii, viii, 2, 4, 13
metabolic pathways, 4
metabolic regulators, vii, 1, 2, 12
metabolic syndrome, vii, viii, 2, 4, 10

metabolism, vii, 1, 2, 4, 5, 7, 8, 9, 10, 12, 13, 15, 89
metabolized, 3
mice, 7, 8, 9, 10, 11, 12, 14, 39
micelles, viii, 17, 18, 25, 26, 29, 30, 31, 32, 34, 38, 40, 41, 43, 44, 45, 49, 50, 51, 52, 53, 54
microbial community(ies), 61, 63, 65, 66, 68, 89, 91, 98
microbiota, 64, 65, 66, 76, 82, 83, 85, 87, 89, 94
microorganisms, 60, 69, 96
microscope, 65
migration, 6, 7, 14
mineralization, 7, 14
mitochondria, 3
mitogen, 11
mixed micelles, vii, viii, 17, 18, 32, 37, 40, 41, 42, 43, 44, 45, 47, 52, 53
mixing, 43
models, 2
molar volume, 32
molecular mass, 35
molecular medicine, 81
molecules, vii, viii, 1, 2, 4, 18, 19, 21, 22, 23, 27, 28, 30, 31, 32, 33, 34, 35, 37, 38, 39, 40, 41, 42, 43, 48, 55, 78
monomers, 18, 27, 28, 30, 40, 41
morbidity, ix, 57, 60, 62, 70, 76, 98
mortality, ix, 57, 60, 61, 70, 76, 83
mortality rate, 76
mRNA, 6
mucin, 15
mucosa, 71
mucus, 60, 62, 64, 67, 69, 97, 98
mucus hypersecretion, 97
mutation, 60

N

NaCl, 25, 27, 49
NAD, 73
NADH, 73
neutral, 3
neutrophils, 62

New England, 98
next generation, 82
nicotinamide, 73
Nissen fundoplication, ix, 58, 80
nitrobenzene, 42
nitrogen, 43
NMR, 30, 51
NPR, 29
nuclear hormone receptor, vii, 1, 2
nuclear magnetic resonance, 52
nuclear receptors, 4, 9, 12, 39

O

obesity, viii, 2, 5, 8, 10, 57, 75
obstruction, 62
obstructive lung disease, 88
oesophageal, ix, 11, 15, 58, 59, 70, 71, 80, 83, 84, 91, 97
oil, 49
opportunities, 81
optimization, 31, 52
organ, 3
organism, 77
outpatient, 80
overlap, 26
overproduction, 69
oxidation, 3, 47, 73
oxygen, 8, 47, 48, 67, 68, 83, 92, 98
oxygen consumption, 8

P

paediatric patients, 60, 64, 81
pain, 71, 81
pancreas, 8
parallel, 19, 30, 38
partition, 24, 44, 46, 50
pathogenesis, 4, 7, 86, 88, 96
pathogens, ix, 57, 58, 61, 62, 63, 67, 69, 74, 75, 76, 77, 78, 79, 81, 91, 94
pathology, ix, 58, 69
pathophysiology, viii, 53, 57, 59, 60, 61, 62, 63, 69, 76, 78, 81, 82

pathway(s), ix, 2, 3, 4, 6, 7, 9, 11, 13, 14, 15, 58, 79, 81
pepsin, 72, 94
peptide, 8, 14, 86
permeability, viii, 11, 18
Perth, 57
pH, 71, 82
pH monitoring, 71
phase diagram, 40, 41
phase transformation, 37, 38
phenotype(s), ix, 58, 76, 79
phosphate, 7, 14
phosphatidylcholine, 54
phosphoenolpyruvate, 6, 7
phospholipids, vii, viii, 17, 18, 32, 38, 48
phosphorylation, 6, 7
phylum, 67, 74
physiological factors, 63
physiology, 53, 81
pilot study, 74
pipeline, 63, 85
placenta, 6
plasma membrane, 6, 54
pneumonia, 61, 70, 73, 98
polar, 18, 25, 32, 37, 41, 55
polar groups, 18
polypeptide, 53
pools, 53
population, ix, 57, 58, 60, 72, 78
prevention, 7, 8, 81
primary micelles, 25, 29, 31, 32
probe, 30
probiotic(s), 67, 76, 90
progenitor cell, 9
prognosis, 68, 81
proliferation, 6, 7, 9, 10, 14, 15
promoter, viii, 12, 15, 18, 32
prostaglandin, 11
proteins, 11, 97
proton pump inhibitors, ix, 58, 86
Pseudomonas aeruginosa, ix, 58, 61, 67, 68, 77, 82, 83, 84, 86, 87, 88, 90, 91, 92, 93, 94, 96, 97, 98
public health, 8, 59

Q

quality of life, ix, 58, 62, 95, 98
quantification, 73, 84

R

radio, 80
radius, 37, 38
reactions, 3
receptor(s), vii, 1, 2, 4, 5, 6, 7, 8, 10, 11, 12, 13, 14, 15, 53, 79, 94
recommendations, 71
recycling, 5
regeneration, viii, 2, 4, 5, 14
rejection, 72
relaxation, 45
relevance, 53
remodelling, 66, 69
repair, 14
repression, 6, 79
repressor, 12
researchers, 32
residue(s), 33, 41, 44
resistance, 12, 39, 50, 55, 89, 91
resolution, 72, 73
respiration, 83
response, 6, 9, 10, 11, 14, 61, 76, 78, 81, 94
responsiveness, 61, 62
restriction fragment length polymorphis, 95
retardation, 49
reticulum, 3
rings, 19, 20, 24, 27
risk, 64, 65, 67, 69, 71, 72, 84
risk factors, 71
RNAs, 92
rods, 40

S

Salmonella, 76, 93, 94
salt concentration, 25, 39, 41, 46

salts, vii, viii, 3, 12, 17, 18, 23, 25, 27, 29, 30, 32, 33, 36, 37, 38, 39, 40, 42, 46, 47, 48, 49, 50, 51, 52, 53, 78, 91, 93

saturation, 41

scattering, 18, 52

secondary micelles, 19, 29, 31

secretion, 2, 5, 8, 10, 14, 39, 42, 54, 59, 62, 77, 79, 83, 84, 92, 93

sedative, 64

sensing, ix, 58, 77, 78, 84, 96

sensitivity, 8, 62, 65, 71, 74, 81

sensor, 4, 76, 92, 94

sequencing, 65, 66, 82, 95

Serbia, 17

serum, 11, 73, 84

shape, 27, 30, 37, 63, 74

sheltered, 18

sibling, 67

side chain, 27

side effects, 81

signal transduction, 11, 81

signaling pathway, 6, 7, 14, 77

signalling, 15

signals, ix, 58, 77, 78, 96

simulation(s), 31, 38, 51, 53

skeletal muscle, 8

skeleton, viii, 17, 19, 20, 21, 22, 23, 24, 25, 26, 27, 29, 31, 33, 37, 38, 41, 42, 48, 51

small intestine, viii, 6, 17

sodium, 25, 30, 31, 35, 36, 38, 42, 50, 51, 52, 53

solubility, 32

solution, 18, 26, 27, 30, 32, 33, 40, 41, 51, 52, 64

species, ix, 54, 58, 65, 66, 67, 68, 69, 76, 78

spectroscopy, 29, 52

sphincter, 59, 71, 80

spin, 30

spleen, 6

Spring, 90

sputum, 63, 64, 65, 68, 72, 73, 74, 78, 83, 92, 93, 95, 97

stability, 31, 43, 85, 86

stabilization, 44

stabilized water molecules, 18

state(s), 37, 43, 44, 54

sterile, 63

steroids, 73

stimulation, 2

stomach, 6, 71, 80

stratification, 74

streptococci, 86

stress response, 7, 14, 90

structure, viii, ix, 17, 18, 25, 31, 32, 36, 38, 40, 50, 52, 53, 58, 66, 68, 83, 91, 94

subjectivity, 72

sulfate, 87

suppression, 77, 79

surfactant, 18, 25, 54

surgical intervention, 80

survival, 76, 91

symbiosis, 94

symmetry, 19

symptoms, ix, 58, 61, 62, 71, 79, 80, 94

synthesis, vii, viii, 2, 3, 4, 5, 6, 11, 12, 48, 88

T

target, 4, 5, 10, 13, 15, 81

taurocholic acid, 3, 39

techniques, 65, 73, 80, 81

technology(ies), 65, 66, 73, 80, 81

temperature, 44, 45

tension, 68

ternary phase diagram, 40, 41

testing, 71

TGR5, vii, 1, 2, 4, 5, 6, 7, 8, 9, 10, 11, 13, 14, 15

therapeutic agents, vii, viii, 2

therapeutics, 59, 81

therapy, 7, 62, 69, 79, 87, 91, 94

thermal energy, 18, 80

thyroid, 4, 8, 13

tissue, 48, 97

tobacco smoke, 59, 60

toxic effect, 46

toxic substances, 59

trade-off, 64

transcription, 6, 10, 12, 15, 53

transcriptomics, 90
transformation, 19, 36, 38
transition to adulthood, 68
translocation, 6
transplant, 72, 84, 85, 91, 95
transplant recipients, 72, 91, 95
transplantation, 72, 73, 95
transport, viii, 2, 17, 32, 39, 46, 53, 54
transportation, 5
trauma, 64
treatment, ix, 6, 7, 8, 13, 58, 66, 68, 71, 79, 80, 81, 83, 86, 87, 89, 90, 91, 92, 94, 97, 98
triggers, 79
tumor, 8
tumor progression, 9
tumorigenesis, 9
type 2 diabetes, 2, 5, 7, 10

U

unforeseen circumstances, 82
uniform, 70
upper respiratory tract, 64, 65
urine, 87

USA, 53, 55

V

validation, 89
vertebrates, viii, 17, 19
very low density lipoprotein, 5, 13
vesicle, 41
vitamins, vii, 1, 2

W

water, 18, 21, 22, 23, 24, 25, 28, 32, 33, 36, 37, 40, 41, 43, 48, 49, 50, 52
World Health Organisation (WHO), 59, 60, 63
worldwide, 59, 60, 62
wound healing, 61

Y

yield, 3, 69